An Introduction
to Fetal Physiology

An Introduction to Fetal Physiology

Frederick C. Battaglia
Giacomo Meschia

*Division of Perinatal Medicine
Department of Pediatrics, Physiology,
and Obstetrics and Gynecology
University of Colorado School of Medicine
Denver, Colorado*

1986

ACADEMIC PRESS, INC.

Harcourt Brace Jovanovich, Publishers

Orlando   San Diego   New York   Austin
Boston   London   Sydney   Tokyo   Toronto

ACADEMIC PRESS, INC.
Orlando, Florida 32887

United Kingdom Edition published by
ACADEMIC PRESS INC. (LONDON) LTD.
24–28 Oval Road, London NW1 7DX

Library of Congress Cataloging in Publication Data

Battaglia, Frederick C., Date
    An introduction to fetal physiology.

    Includes index.
    1. Fetus—Physiology.   I. Meschia, Giacomo.
II. Title.
RG610.B37   1986   612'.647   86-10757
ISBN 0—12—081920—1 (alk. paper)

PRINTED IN THE UNITED STATES OF AMERICA

86 87 88 89   9 8 7 6 5 4 3 2 1

Contents

4 FETAL AND PLACENTAL METABOLISM: PART II. AMINO ACIDS AND LIPIDS   100

5 INDIVIDUAL ORGAN METABOLISM IN THE FETUS   136

6 FETAL RESPIRATORY PHYSIOLOGY   154

Preface

In the last twenty years the study of fetal physiology has generated a substantial body of data. Since the quantity and variety of these data can be a major challenge for the student struggling to identify basic concepts, we have attempted to organize and critically evaluate some of the new information with the intent of producing an introductory text which would be of general interest to physiologists as well as to faculty, residents, and postdoctoral fellows in obstetrics and pediatrics.

We have not attempted to produce a text in which data (often conflicting) collected in all spheres of fetal and placental physiology are presented because we believe that this is better done through publications in which several authors contribute their specialized knowledge. Rather we have presented information which supports the establishment of concepts in fetal physiology. In large part this approach reflects the influence that Professor Donald H. Barron had on our thinking. We owe a great debt to him for his patience as a teacher, and we have fond memories of the many hours spent in his office at Yale School of Medicine discussing Sir Joseph Barcroft's approach to physiology, an approach which Donald Barron carried forward. His work led to the development of biologic preparations permitting a study of fetal physiology under comparatively "normal" conditions. In that environment we could not fail to be impressed with the importance of searching for the broad implications and logical coherence of physiological data.

The beginnings of fetal physiology are rooted in measurements of placental and fetal growth and in comparative studies of placental histology that were made long before physiologic data could be collected and properly understood. In the first chapter we review this evidence, both to lay a foundation for the succeeding chapters and to demonstrate how newly acquired knowledge is changing our perception of what that evidence means. The second chapter develops a conceptual basis for the physiology of placental exchange. The next three chapters introduce the reader to present knowledge of fetal and placental metabolism. In these chapters we have included a discussion of methodological issues, because a fair amount of misinformation about fetal metabolism can be traced to the use of faulty methodology and/or difficulties in the correct interpretation of what has been measured. The sixth and seventh chapters are an introduction to fetal respiratory and circulatory physiology with emphasis on the integration and meaning of factual information. Finally, the last two chapters present a brief summary of current knowledge about uteroplacental blood flow regulation and fetal water balance.

Throughout this book we have focused attention upon a comparative approach, because perinatal biology encompasses marked differences among mammals in placentation, in fetal and neonatal development, and in the adaptations made by the mother during pregnancy and lactation. These interspecies differences have led investigators on occasion to approach the variability among species as a difficulty which must be overcome in searching for a perfect "animal model" of human fetal physiology. We hope this book emphasizes how a study of the way in which different species solve the common problem of producing a viable offspring can bring out concepts in perinatal biology which bridge interspecies differences.

We would like to take this opportunity to acknowledge our indebtedness to our teachers, friends, and collaborators. In addition to Dr. D. H. Barron, two of our teachers deserve special thanks: Rodolfo Margaria (G. M.) and Robert E. Cooke (F. C. B.). We are most grateful to all the investigators whose work forms the basis of this book and in particular to Edgar L. Makowski for many years of happy and fruitful collaboration.

Frederick C. Battaglia
Giacomo Meschia

An Introduction
to Fetal Physiology

1

Fetal and Placental Growth

MASS OF THE FETUS

In all species, fetal weight tends to increase exponentially for at least part of gestation. In humans, the birthweights of infants delivered at different gestational ages follow a growth curve in which fetal weight increases exponentially until the latter part of gestation, when fetal growth rate slows leading to a typical S-shaped curve of newborn weight versus gestational age (9). There is an apparent conflict between these observations generated by birthweight information and those obtained in recent years which have used repeated estimates of fetal size in the same pregnant woman by means of ultrasonic techniques. Such ultrasonic measurements of human fetal growth have suggested that there is a constant rate of growth in late gestation with no apparent "slowing" near term. The reasons for these different conclusions drawn from birthweight information versus ultrasonic studies are not yet clear. The conflict may in part reflect that even the best ultrasonic estimates of fetal size would have errors of ±10%. Differences in describing fetal growth as constant or decelerating over the last few weeks of gestation cannot be easily established by a methodology with a large variance in the measurement of fetal size.

In sheep, a semilogarithmic plot of fetal weight versus gestational age does not yield a straight line but instead gives a curve with convexity toward the weight axis (Figure 1-1), indicating that the fractional rate of

1

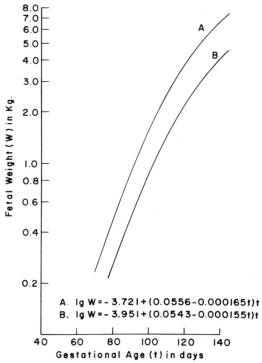

Figure 1-1: Semilogarithmic plot of fetal growth curves in two breeds of sheep that produce lambs with different birth weights. Curve A drawn from data by Koong et al. (20). Curve B from data in authors' laboratory.

weight gain is greater in early pregnancy. Several equations (the equations in Figure 1-1 are examples) have been derived for the purpose of mathematically defining the "fetal growth curve." Although useful from a descriptive viewpoint, such equations do not have a precise, theoretical meaning because of the complex changes in fetal body composition during pregnancy (see below) that preclude any simple interpretation of fetal growth.

At the end of gestation, fetal mass varies considerably among mammals reflecting both differences in fetal growth rate and differences in gestation length. If one includes the marsupials, the range in newborn weight from the smallest marsupial weighing 10 mg to the largest eutherian mammal—the blue whale, weighing 2000 kg—is 200 million-fold. Figure 1-2 is reproduced from Tyndale–Biscoe's text and illustrates the range in newborn weights among marsupials (34). Even the newborn of the largest marsupi-

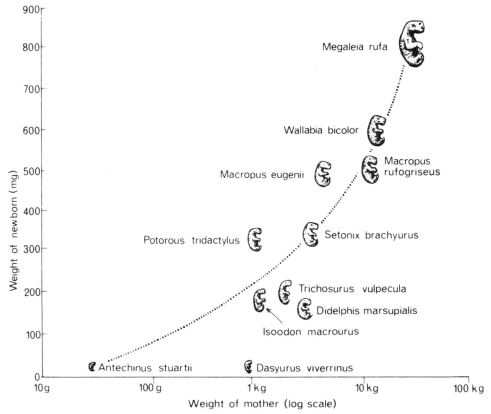

Figure 1-2: Relationship of newborn weight to maternal weight in marsupials (34).

als only attain a weight of approximately 750 mg; for example, even in the 40 kg red kangaroo, the newborn weight does not equal 1 g. Some of the marsupials have a large litter size which does not, however, make up for the very small size of individual fetuses. From the fact that the total fetal mass (i.e., fetal weight × litter size) may still represent less than 0.1% maternal body weight, it would seem likely that pregnancy presents relatively little metabolic demand upon the marsupial mother, whereas lactation would impose a far greater stress. By contrast, eutherian mammals have a tendency to produce a relatively large fetal mass. This is especially true for small eutherian mammals. Figure 1-3 is based on a set of data collected by Leitch *et al.* (23) and demonstrates quite clearly the inverse relationship between *total* newborn weight, expressed as percentage of maternal weight, and animal size. It also demonstrates the remarkable

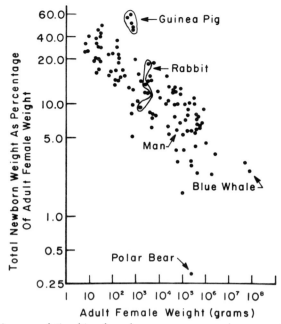

Figure 1-3: Inverse relationship of newborn mass, expressed as percentage of maternal mass, and adult animal size. In this figure newborn mass for polytocous species is the weight of all the fetuses in a litter. Drawn from data by Leitch *et al.* (23).

differences in the amount of fetal mass produced by mammals of comparable size.

It is well known that the primates, including humans, produce a relatively small fetal mass in relation to the duration of pregnancy (6, 18). In an attempt to present a unifying hypothesis for the great differences in fetal growth rate among mammals, Sacher and Staffeldt (28) proposed the hypothesis that "Rates of fetal growth in mammals are governed by a common limiting factor, the rate of growth of neural tissue." While there is still considerable variability in brain growth rate among mammals (the range is approximately $0.015–0.033$ $g^{1/3}$/day), there is considerably less variability than in the fetal body growth rate which varies from 0.033 to 0.25 $g^{1/3}$/day. The physiological basis for the correlation of brain weight and gestation time is unknown. By contrast, we shall demonstrate in subsequent chapters that considerable progress has been made in defining those aspects of metabolism and placental function that underlie the variability in newborn: maternal mass ratio among mammals. Physiological data suggest the concept that in the course of mammalian evolution prob-

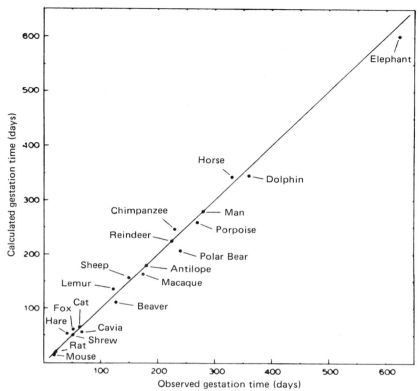

Figure 1-4:   Comparison between the estimated gestation time ($G_{calc} = 26 \, L^{-0.6}\bar{E}_n^{0.06}P_a^{0.183}$) and the actual recorded gestation time (G_{obs}) in mammals. L = litter size; $\bar{E}_n$ = mean neonatal brain weight (g); P_a = adult body weight of nonpregnant female (g). G_{calc} has been tested for a sample of 20 species of placental mammals ($r = 0.996$) (17).

lems of oxygen and nutrient supply played an important role in limiting the growth of fetal metabolic demand. Given this concept, Hofman (17) has pointed out that the intrauterine development of a large brain : body mass ratio in humans is favored by a gestation with a single fetus and is made possible by a slow rate of fetal somatic growth. The latter allows steady increase in fetal cerebral metabolic demand while the total metabolic demand of the conceptus is kept within viable limits. The interrelationships of brain size, litter size, and maternal body weight in determining gestation length is summarized in Figure 1-4 from Hofman's study (17). It is clear that the length of gestation can be reasonably well predicted by the weighting given each of the above factors.

The fetal and placental metabolic demand has two components: (a) the fetal and placental accretion of organic matter in the form of new tissue, fat, and glycogen stores; and (b) the fetal and placental uptake of substrates used for energy metabolism. Both demands can be expressed in units of energy (that is, in calories or joules) and compared with maternal energy requirements. We shall discuss fetal and placental energy metabolism in Chapter 3. In this next section, we consider the relationship of fetal growth to fetal caloric accretion.

FETAL BODY COMPOSITION

In considering fetal growth from a metabolic viewpoint, the body composition of the fetus can be broken down into three major components: water, fat, and nonfat dry weight.

Water

Since this component has no caloric value, it must be considered whenever the metabolic implications of fetal weight changes are discussed. In all species, fetal body water, expressed as a percentage of body weight, decreases with increasing gestation. This is illustrated in Figure 1-5 which compares the decline in fetal body water for four species (5, 30, 35). Part C of the figure illustrates the fact that fetal body water tends to decrease

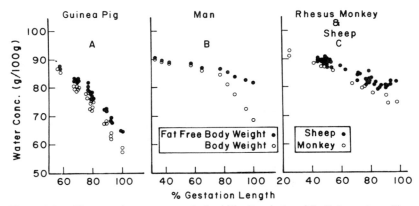

Figure 1-5: Changes of water content in fetal life. Panels A and B: Guinea pig and human fetal water content, expressed as a percentage of body weight and as a percentage of fat-free body weight. Panel C: Fetal water content as a percentage of body weight in the sheep and rhesus monkey, two species in which there is a relatively small accumulation of fat during fetal life.

fairly linearly for species with little fetal body fat, such as monkey and sheep. In parts A and B, water is expressed both as a percentage of body weight and as a percentage of fat free body weight for the data from guinea pigs and from humans. Since there is a large concentration of fat which accumulates during fetal life in these two species, the concentration of water in the fetal body is further diluted as fat accretion accelerates in late gestation. The changes in water content during gestation are particularly important for their impact upon the interpretation of weight-specific metabolic rate. Although wet weight is a convenient and sometimes appropriate standard, other references such as dry weight and fat-free dry weight must be considered for the proper interpretation of fetal metabolic data. Studies in various species suggest that extracellular water as a percentage of body weight decreases more than intracellular water as gestation advances (8). On an absolute scale, both extra- and intracellular water volumes are increasing as gestation advances, but as a concentration of body components, both phases are decreasing.

Fat

Fat represents the fetal component with the greatest variability among mammalian species. This is of particular significance when we recall that fat has a very high energy content, 9.5 kcal/g, and a very high carbon content, approximately 78%. Thus, differences in fetal fat concentration among species lead to large differences in the calculated caloric accretion rates and in the carbon requirements of the fetal tissues for growth.

Nonfat Dry Weight

This category represents the residual composition of the fetal tissues. If this material is further analyzed for its total amino acid content, then it can be subdivided into the protein and the nonfat, nonprotein dry weight.

The caloric values of each of these three components are presented in Table 1-1. In any calculation of the caloric accretion rate of fetal tissues, it is not strictly necessary to separate the nonfat dry weight into protein and nonprotein components. The reason for this is apparent in Table 1-1. The caloric concentration of the nonfat dry weight seems to be fairly consistent across species and also within species at different developmental stages, implying that the proportion of protein to nonprotein in the tissues is approximately the same. For these reasons the caloric accretion rate of any fetus or newborn can be estimated from the growth curve of the species and the changing fat and water concentrations.

Table 1-1

Energy Value of Tissue Components

Tissue component	Energy value (kcal/g)[a]
H$_2$O	0
Fat	9.45
Nonfat dry weight	
Pig	4.0–4.6 (10)
Lamb	4.4–4.6 (27)
Guinea pig	4.6 (30)
Carbohydrate	4.15
	(3.7–4.2)
Protein	5.65
In vivo catabolism	4.35

[a] 1 kcal = 4190 J.

For example, Table 1-2 presents the caloric distribution for a term newborn infant. Since the term newborn infant has a high concentration of white fat depots, the caloric concentration of the infant's weight is quite high (30, 35, 36). The overall importance of fat in determining caloric accretion rates is evident from the fact that its caloric density is more than 12 times that of the nonfat wet weight (9.45 versus 0.75 kcal/g). While fat represents approximately 61% of the caloric value of the term infant, it represents an even larger percentage of the calories deposited each day in the new tissue, since in late gestation the rate of fat accretion is greater than the nonfat accretion rate. The significance of a changing caloric distribution within the new tissue built each day was brought out in a study describing the rate of caloric accretion for the human fetus (30). Figure 1-6 taken from that report illustrates that an increasingly large fraction of the caloric accretion of the human fetus over the period of neonatal viability, 26 weeks to term, is represented by fat. For any species, the caloric accretion at two different times in development, T_1 and T_2

Table 1-2

Calculation of the Caloric Distribution in the Term Human Infant[a]

	Wet weight	Fat	Nonfat wet weight	Nonfat dry weight
Weight (g)	3450	386	3064	511
Total calories (kcal)	5950	3650	2300	2300
Caloric concentration (kcal/g)	1.72	9.45	0.75	4.5

[a] The values in this table are from Ziegler *et al.* (36).

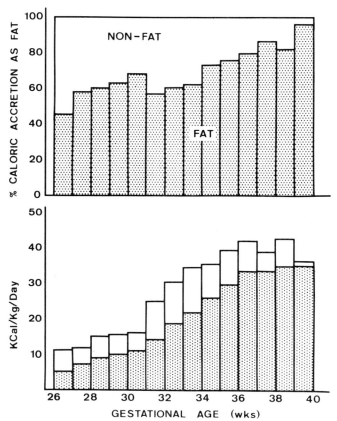

Figure 1-6: Estimated caloric accretion in the human fetus during the last 14 weeks of pregnancy. Upper panel: Contribution of fat to total caloric accretion. Lower panel: Daily fat and nonfat caloric accretion per kilogram of body weight. Reproduced from Sparks *et al.* (30) by permission of S. Karger AG, Basel.

(defining a sufficiently short interval so that an assumption of linear changes in wet weight and in concentrations of fat and water is reasonable) can be estimated as follows:

Caloric accretion
In nonfat tissues: [(wet wgt fat and $H_2O)T_2$ − (wet wgt fat and $H_2O)T_1$] × 4.5
In fat tissues: [(fat content)T_2 − (fat content)T_1] × 9.45
Sum of caloric accretion

In the latter part of gestation in humans the fetus is growing at approximately 1.5%/day or 15 g/kg/day. The nonfat dry weight increases approximately 2.25 g/kg/day. However, the rate of fat accretion is more variable. In a normally developing fetus approximately 3.5 g/kg/day of fat would be added to the 2.25 g of nonfat dry weight, the remainder of the 15 g representing water accretion. From the caloric values give in Table 1-1, fetal caloric accretion rate in humans can be calculated to be the following:

$$
\begin{aligned}
\text{For non-fat dry weight: } & 2.25 \times 4.5 \ \ = 10.12 \\
\text{For fat: } & \underline{3.5 \ \ \times 9.45 = 33.07} \\
& 43.19
\end{aligned}
$$

Since the energy metabolism of the human fetus has been estimated at approximately 50 kcal/kg/day, it follows that for an infant not accumulating fat at an appreciable rate, the growth of nonfat tissues could be maintained with a placental supply of nutrients equal to 50 + 10 kcal/kg/day. However, it should be emphasized that accretion of new tissue without fat is not a normal process in the human fetus and newborn. Similar calculations could be made in other species given the body composition and accretion rates in the species.

PLACENTAL MORPHOLOGY

Embryos develop a highly vascularized membrane, the chorion, which functions to mediate the exchange of heat and matter with the maternal organism. The chorionic epithelium (trophoblast) comes in contact and interacts with maternal tissues to form a structure which is referred to as the "placental barrier" or "placental membrane." The formation and histology of the placental membrane are markedly different among mammals.

In 1909 Grosser (15) proposed a classification which uses the maternal tissue with which the outer surface of the chorion is in contact as the distinguishing characteristic of the placental barrier. According to Grosser's criteria, there are three major types of placental membranes.

Epitheliochorial

The placental membrane is formed by apposition of the chorion to the epithelium of the uterine mucosa. Well described examples of this type of membrane are found in the equine, porcine, ovine, and bovine placentas. Figure 1-7 shows an example of the epitheliochorial type of placental

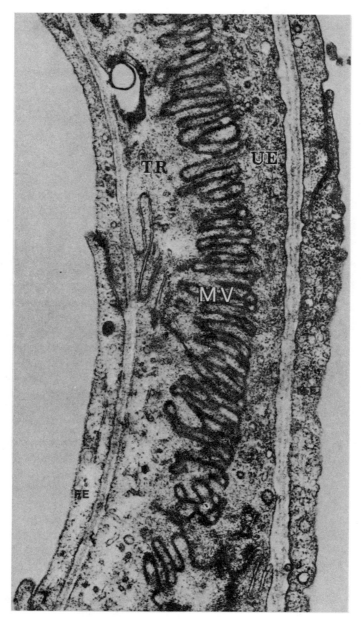

Figure 1-7: Placental barrier in the epitheliochorical placenta of the pig. The main tissue layers interposed between fetal and maternal blood are the fetal endothelium (FE), the trophoblast (TR), the uterine epithelium (UE), and the maternal endothelium (ME). The maternal and fetal epithelial surfaces have microvilli (MV) that interdigitate (×32,400) (13).

barrier (13). In the past the placentas of sheep and cattle were not classified as epitheliochorial, but as syndesmochorial, because with light microscopy alone the chorionic surface was thought to be in direct contact with the connective tissues of the uterine mucosa. Electron microscopic studies have corrected this misconception.

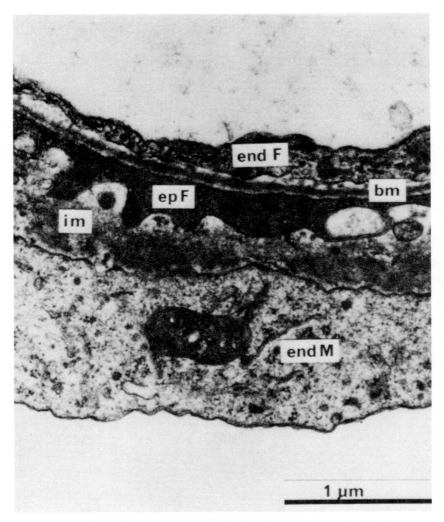

Figure 1-8: Placental barrier in the endotheliochorial placenta of the dog. The tissue layers interposed between fetal and maternal blood are the fetal endothelium (end F), the basement membranes of fetal endothelium and chorionic epithelium (ep F) fused into a single lamina (bm), the maternal interstitium (im), and the maternal endothelium (end M) (32).

Endotheliochorial

The placental membrane is formed by apposition of the chorion to the endothelium of the maternal capillaries. The best known examples of this type are in the placentas of carnivores. Figure 1-8 presents the histology of the placental barrier in dogs (32).

Hemochorial

In some mammals, including rodents and most primates, the chorion invades the stroma of the uterine mucosa, destroys the endometrial capillaries, and comes in direct contact with maternal blood. Figure 1-9 shows the histology of the hemochorial barrier in the human placenta.

In the 1950s, Flexner and Gellhorn (11) made a comparative study of the permeability of the placental barrier to tracer sodium and concluded that there was an excellent correlation between Grosser's classification of placental types and placental permeability, the epitheliochorial variety being the least permeable and the hemochorial being the most permeable. These findings seemed to validate the hypothesis, which was prevalent at the time, that Grosser's classification groups together placentas which are similar in all important aspects of placental transfer. Furthermore, a common inference grew out of such observations, namely, that the human

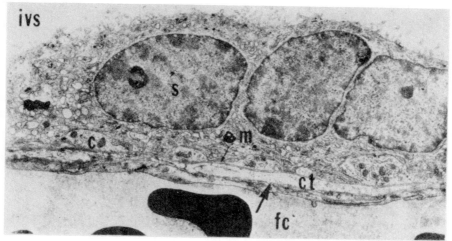

Figure 1-9: Placental barrier in the hemochorial human placenta at term. Maternal blood in the intervillous space (ivs) is separated from fetal blood in the fetal capillaries (fc) by the trophoblastic epithelium, which is composed of syncytial trophoblast (s) and cytotrophoblast (c), some fetal connective tissue (ct), and the endothelium of the fetal capillaries. The light and heavy arrows point to the trophoblastic basement membrane and the basement membrane of the fetal endothelium, respectively. A myeloid figure (m), indicative of degeneration, is shown in the trophoblast (9a; courtesy of Dr. Ralph Wynn).

placenta is the most "efficient" type of placenta. However, subsequent studies have thoroughly disproved the validity of this hypothesis. With reference to problems of placental transfer, there are important differences among placentas within a group, as well as important similarities among placentas of different groups, none of which could be predicted on the basis of Grosser's (15) scheme. Without attempting to make this subject unnecessarily complex, it is sufficient to note that the placental transfer of any given molecule depends upon many different properties of the placenta, such as rate of maternal and fetal placental blood flows; the pattern of placental perfusion (whether concurrent, countercurrent or otherwise); the surface, thickness, and physicochemical properties of the placental membrane; the metabolic activity of the placenta; the various mechanisms of transfer which are available (e.g., diffusion, carrier mediated transfer, active transfer); and regional differences within a placenta in placental histology and function. For the hypothesis to be valid, there should be a correlation between the histology of the placental membrane, as defined by Grosser, and all those other aspects of placental structure which are relevant to placental transfer. Such a correlation is missing, which becomes apparent if we consider two aspects of placental morphology: a comparative morphometric study of the placental villous surface by Baur (3) and the histology of the placental circulation.

According to Baur's study, there is a fundamental difference between compact and diffuse placentas. In compact placentas the placental villi develop only in certain specialized areas of the chorionic sac to form compact, macroscopically distinct structures (e.g., placental cotyledons), whereas in diffuse placentas the villi are distributed over the whole chorion, the placenta itself assuming the macroscopic appearance of a membrane covering the inner surface of the uterine wall. The villous surface of compact placentas at term is well correlated to fetal weight from rat to elephant, irrespective of the position of each placenta in Grosser's classification (Figure 1-10). Among diffuse placentas there is also a correlation between villous surfaces and fetal weight, but at comparable fetal weights diffuse placentas have approximately seven times less villous surface than the compact placentas. Although the functional meaning of the large difference in surface area between compact and diffuse placentas is not clear, it is likely to be as important physiologically as the number of tissue layers interposed between maternal and fetal blood.

HISTOLOGY OF THE PLACENTAL VASCULAR BED

The histologic study of placental vascularization is technically difficult. For this reason relatively few species have been investigated and some major issues remain unresolved. Nevertheless, the present knowledge is

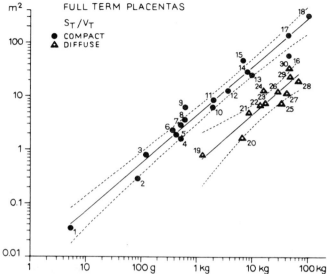

Figure 1-10: Villous surface area (S_T), plotted in logarithmic coordinates against the sum of placental and fetal weight (V_T). The dashed lines show the 95% confidence limits of the two regression lines for compact and diffuse placentas. Compact placentas: 1 rat, 2 guinea pig (*Cavia*), 3 cat, 4 German sheep dog, 5 sloth (*Choloepus didactylus*), 6 crab-eating monkey (*Macaca fascicularis*), 7 douc langur (*Pygathrix nemea*), 8 Guereza (*Colobus polycomos*), 9 leopard, 10 chimpanzee, 11 gorilla, 12 human, 13 dwarf zebu, 14 seal (*Phoea vitulina*), 15 sea lion (*Zalophus californianus*), 16 giraffe (*Giraffa camelopardalis tippelskirchi*), 17 European domestic cow, and 18 African elephant. Diffuse placentas: 19 European domestic pig, 20 dwarf hippopotamus (*Choeropsis liberiensis*), 21 dolphin, 22 llama, 23 pony, 24 Sardinian dwarf donkey, 25 zebra, 26 Somalian wild ass (*Asinus asinus somalicus*), 27 Bactrian camel, 28 Indian rhinoceros (*Rh. unicornis*), 29 horse (thoroughbred), and 30 hippopotamus (*H. amphibicus*) (3).

sufficient to establish the concept that there are major interspecies differences, which are as pronounced as differences in the histology of the placental barrier and do not correlate with the differences emphasized by Grosser's classification. In some species the maternal and fetal placental circulations form a highly efficient, countercurrent exchange system, whereas in other species the two circulations form a much less efficient exchanger, which we have called *venous equilibrator* (see Chapter 2).

Let us consider first the differences within two epitheliochorial placentas, those of the horse and of the sheep. In the epitheliochorial placenta of the horse there are thousands of small globular structures, each 1–2 mm in diameter, which are called *microcotyledons* (29). Maternal arteries run outside each microcotyledon and reach the epithelium of the uterine mucosa (Figure 1-11). Here they form branches that penetrate the cotyledon beneath its fetal surface and give rise to a capillary network that perfuses the maternal side of the placental barrier. Venous channels drain this network and direct the flow of blood toward the base of the cotyledon. On the fetal side of the barrier, blood is carried to the tip of short chorionic villi by arterioles located in the center of each villus and then flows back to the base of the villus via a capillary network and is collected by venules that return it to the fetus. From the physiologic point of view, the important aspect of this description is the suggestion that within the cotyledon, maternal and fetal blood run in opposite directions.

In sheep, placental cotyledons are formed by interaction of the chorion with highly vascularized areas of the uterine mucosa which are known as *caruncles*. Thus, the number of cotyledons that can be formed is limited by the fact that there are approximately 100 caruncles, evenly distributed in the two horns of the uterus. In the case of twins, each fetus has approximately 50 caruncles available for implantation. The fully developed sheep cotyledon is a large structure which weighs approximately 5 g. Inside each cotyledon the epitheliochorial surface is folded to form villi. Maternal arteries enter the maternal surface of the cotyledon and run toward the fetal surface, giving off branches which tend to be at right

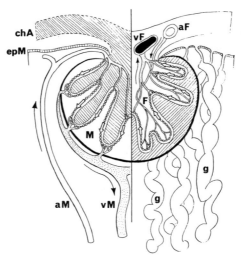

Figure 1-11: Diagram showing the arrangement of maternal and fetal blood vessels in the microcotyledons of the equine placenta. Small open arrows demonstrate the postulated countercurrent directions of maternal and fetal blood flows. aM, maternal artery; vM, maternal vein; chA, chorioallantois; epM, uterine epithelium; g, endometrial glands; aF, fetal artery; vF, fetal vein; F, fetal; M, maternal. Based on data by Tsutsumi (33); reproduced with permission from Ref. 29.

angles to the main vessel. On the fetal side, each villus has a central arteriole which gives off relatively few branches before reaching the tip of the villus. Morphologic studies attempting to define the relative direction of maternal and fetal blood in the ovine placenta have not provided a definitive answer. Although it is clear that the system cannot be described as a countercurrent exchanger, the actual pattern of maternal and fetal perfusion may be too complex to allow for any simple morphologic definition. However, such placentas as the sheep placenta can still be usefully characterized by their functional properties. With regard to placental oxygen transfer, a type of function in which the pattern of placental perfusion plays an important role, the horse and sheep placenta have markedly different properties (see Chapter 6). The horse placenta demonstrates some of the properties of a countercurrent exchanger, whereas the sheep placenta demonstrates the properties of a venous equilibrator.

Within the hemochorial group of placentas, two distinct circulatory patterns have been described, one exemplified by the placenta of small rodents and rabbits and the other by the human placenta. Figure 1-12 shows a schematic representation of the rabbit placenta (7). Maternal

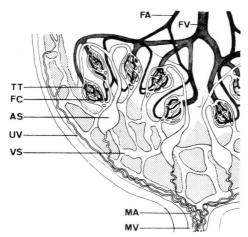

Figure 1-12: Diagram showing the arrangement of maternal and fetal blood vessels in the rabbit placenta. The decidual portion of the placenta is stippled and the trophoblastic portion unstippled. Maternal blood enters the exchange area via arteries (MA) that feed large arterial sinuses (AS). Efferent arteries proceed from these sinuses toward the fetal surface of the placenta and open into the trophoblastic tubules (TT) of the placental labyrinth. In these tubules the blood flows toward the decidua, where it collects in venous sinuses (VS) that are drained by large veins in the uterine wall (UV) and mesometrium (MV). The fetal arteries (FA) penetrate deep into the placenta and then break up into capillaries (FC) in which fetal blood runs back toward the fetal umbilical veins (FV). Based on an original drawing by Mossman (24). From Carter (7).

arteries which arise from large arterial sinuses run toward the fetal surface of the placenta where they subdivide into several branches. From these branches the maternal blood turns inward and flows through capillarylike tubules of trophoblast known as the *labyrinth*. On the other side of the placental barrier, fetal arteries carry blood directly to the maternal end of the labyrinth, from which it flows back to the fetus through a network of capillaries. The important aspect of this arrangement is that in the exchange area (the labyrinth), maternal and fetal blood run in opposite directions.

In the human placenta the chorion forms villi resembling a grove of trees instead of forming a labyrinth (Figure 1-13) (26). Each tree stems from the fetal surface of the placenta and immerses its branches in a pool of maternal blood known as the intervillus space. In the mature human placenta there are approximately 200 such trees. Some branches float freely in the space and some are anchored either to the maternal surface of the placenta (basal plate) or to septa which arise from this surface and subdivide the organ into cotyledons. In marked contrast to the placenta of rodents and rabbits, the maternal arteries do not extend to the fetal surface of the placenta but terminate at the basal plate. Maternal blood is ejected into the intervillus space from the arterial openings in the basal

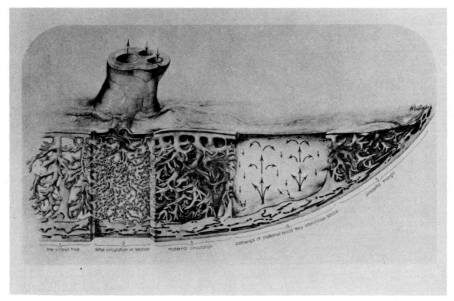

Figure 1-13: Diagram showing the circulation of maternal and fetal blood in the human placenta according to Ramsey (26).

plate and is drained through venous openings which are also located on the maternal surface of the intervillus space. The absence of any capillaries or capillarylike channels in the maternal circulation of the human placenta presents a difficulty in visualizing the path of maternal blood as it runs through the intervillus space. Two different descriptions have been put forward.

According to one description (Figure 1-13) (26), the dense arborization of the fetal villi is evenly distributed in the intervillus space. Arterial blood is ejected under pressure against the terminal branches of this arborization and forms a conical jet directed toward the chorionic plate. The villi and the walls of the intervillus space reflect the ejected blood back toward the venous openings. According to a second description (12), the chorionic villi do not grow evenly in the intervillus space but leave an empty space in front of the arterial openings. Maternal blood enters this hollow space first and then it is dispersed laterally through the arborization of the villi. Freese has produced *in vivo* evidence that could be explained by this type of circulatory arrangement (12). Contrast medium injected into the arterial system of a pregnant monkey rapidly entered the placenta, creating circles of fairly uniform opacity around the entry sites of arterial blood. A few seconds after the injection, the opacity began to disappear from the center of each circle, which acquired the appearance of a smoke ring.

The marked histological differences in the circulation of the labyrinthine-hemochorial and the villous-hemochorial placenta have functional significance. As explained in subsequent chapters, the placentas of guinea pigs and rabbits function like countercurrent exchangers, whereas the level of performance of the human placenta appears to be that of a venous equilibrator.

To summarize our discussion of placental morphology, it is evident that no single attribute of placental structure is sufficient for the purpose of classifying placental types. For example, in comparing the placenta of any given mammal to the human placenta, we should compare the histology of the placental barrier (is the placenta hemochorial?), the surface area (is the placenta compact or diffuse?), and the perfusion pattern (what is the relative direction of maternal and fetal placental blood flows?). Each of these properties is important with respect to some aspect of placental function and does not covary with the other properties.

PLACENTAL GROWTH AND MATURATION

Placental growth and maturation can be addressed from several viewpoints. There are those characteristics of placentation that are common to all mammals; there are the special characteristics of each species; and finally, there are the linkages between placentation on the one hand and maternal or fetal physiologic changes on the other hand. One of the most important questions is how changes in placental size and function relate to changes in fetal metabolic demands. Note that this question is similar to that posed in postnatal life for the relationship of lung development to oxygen requirements of a growing organism (14, 19).

In general, placental development involves three stages: implantation, growth, and maturation. It is clear that events occurring at the time of implantation play a role in determining the ultimate size attained by the placenta. This conclusion is based on studies in species where potential implantation sites can be identified prior to implantation. These preimplantation sites, or "caruncles," are present in the sheep uterus. Some years ago Alexander (1, 2) was able to show that the smaller the number of caruncles that are available for the formation of placental cotyledons, the smaller the placental weight at term. He also demonstrated an inverse relationship between the average cotyledonary weight and the number of implantation sites. Thus, there is some compensatory growth of individual cotyledons when their total number is reduced.

By approximately the fiftieth day of gestation in the sheep, the implantation phase is complete and the total cotyledonary number has reached its maximum. The placenta then enters a rapid growth phase which is completed at approximately the ninetieth day of gestation. From then until term (145 days), placental weight and DNA content do not increase (placental weight actually decreases) while fetal weight continues its exponential increase. In sheep the placental cotyledons weigh approximately three times as much as the fetus at mid-gestation and one-tenth of the fetal weight at term. In the past, the progressive, large increase in the fetal : placental mass ratio during gestation was misinterpreted as a reflection of a limitation in placental function that develops as the fetus "outgrows" its placenta. The concept that the term placenta is an "aging organ" stems in part from this theory. The assumption that during pregnancy there is a progressive decline in the ability of the placenta to supply oxygen and nutrients to the growing fetus is incorrect because it does not take into account the last phase of placental development. This last phase is the functional maturation which occurs in this organ at a time when placental size and total DNA content are no longer increasing. Both morphometric and physiologic data have demonstrated this maturation process. It should be emphasized that the differences in placental growth patterns among species do not alter these general conclusions. For example, the human placenta shows a progressive increase in weight until term but not nearly in proportion to the rapid increase in fetal weight, and, just

as in the sheep, the fetal : placental ratio increases as gestation progresses.

FUNCTIONAL MATURATION OF THE PLACENTA

Morphometric studies of the placenta in a relatively large number of
species have shown that the surface area of the placental villi (i.e., the
villous surface area that is visible under light microscopy) continues to
increase throughout gestation (Figure 1-14) (3). This observation implies
that the growth of the surface across which the maternal-fetal metabolic
exchange takes place is synchronized with the growth of fetal metabolic
demands. In addition to an increase in surface area, the thickness of the
placental barrier decreases with gestation. For example, in the human
placenta the cytotrophoblast tends to disappear and the syncytiotrophoblast thins markedly.

In agreement with morphometric evidence, physiological studies have
demonstrated that placental urea diffusing capacity (i.e., permeability)
increases throughout pregnancy in the sheep, even in the second half of
gestation when placental growth has ended (21). Thus, if urea permeability is expressed per gram of placenta (or per gram of placental DNA),
there is a striking increase in the last third of gestation, as illustrated in
Figure 1-15, upper panel. The permeability of the placental membrane to

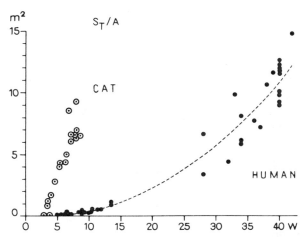

Figure 1-14:   Growth of the surface area of the placental membrane in cats (dotted circles)
and humans (full circles). The surface area in square meters is plotted against gestational age in
weeks (3).

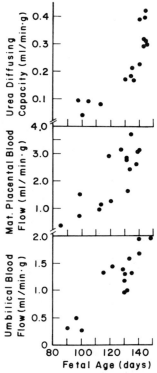

Figure 1-15: Functional maturation of the placenta in sheep. From 80 to 140 days placental urea diffusing capacity, maternal placental blood flow, and umbilical blood flow per gram of placenta increase markedly.

urea depends upon its area and is inversely related to its thickness (see Chapter 2). Concomitant with the increase in placental permeability, there is also an increase in maternal and fetal placental blood flows indicating a maturation of several important aspects of placental function (Figure 1-15, lower panels). The capacity of the term placenta to support fetal growth is also documented by the observations in rabbits that pregnancy can be prolonged with appropriate endocrine treatment and that the fetuses of such prolonged pregnancies are markedly increased in size without a significant increase in placental weight (16).

Numerous studies in several species have attempted to define the relationship and interdependence of fetal and placental weight. As we have seen, no meaningful relationship could be established by comparing placentas and fetuses of different ages. Both the "functional value" of 1 g of placenta and fetal body composition change continuously during preg-

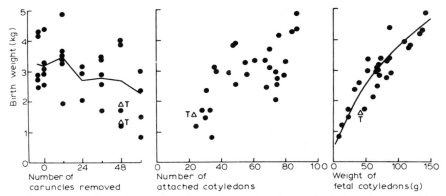

Figure 1-16: Effect of surgically reducing the number of caruncles in the ovine uterus. Birth weight was inversely related to the number of caruncles removed and showed a positive correlation with the number and weight of the placental cotyledons that were formed after carunclectomy. T, data on twins (2).

nancy. Therefore, one cannot pool data about placentas and fetuses that are different in age as well as in size. By contrast, studies limited to a narrow window of gestational age have demonstrated a positive and significant correlation between placental and fetal weight. It would seem that a small placenta can restrain fetal growth. The hypothesis that fetal growth retardation can be secondary to stunted placental growth has some support from experimental evidence. First, in the carunculectomy experiments by Alexander (1, 2) there was a high incidence of fetal growth retardation and a strong correlation between placental and fetal weight (Figure 1-16). Because growth retardation was obtained in this case by interfering with the process of implantation, it seems likely that the primary effect of the experimental procedure was to stunt placental growth and that the stunting of fetal growth was secondary to a deficiency of placental function. Second, there is evidence that in growth-retarded fetuses associated with a small placenta, there is an imbalance between placental function and fetal metabolic demands. In eight term lamb fetuses ranging in weight from 2.4 to 5.4 kg, placental urea permeability per kilogram of fetus spanned a wide range from 11 to 31 ml/kg/min of fetus. However, placental size and total DNA content also varied, and there was a close correlation between permeability per kilogram of fetus and placental DNA content (Figure 1-17) (21). These observations suggest that in a fetus with a small placenta, the area of maternal-fetal exchange is small, not only in absolute terms, but more importantly, in relation to fetal metabolic demands.

There are probably many factors that regulate the growth of the placen-

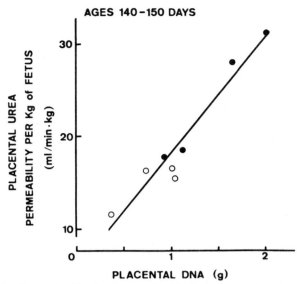

Figure 1-17:   Among fetal lambs of approximately the same age, there is a positive correlation between urea permeability per kilogram of fetus and total placental DNA. O, singletons; ●, twins (21).

tal membrane and the placental vasculature. In the rhesus monkey, if the fetus is removed by caesarean section, the placenta is retained even beyond term but stops growing in size. The syncytiotrophoblast continues to secrete placental lactogen and shows the persistence of an abundant endoplasmic reticulum for up to 2 months after fetectomy (22, 25). However, the fetal capillaries degenerate and the cytotrophoblast disappears. These results suggest that placental growth and the maintenance of some of the placental tissues depend upon the continuous supply of trophic factors by the fetus. Unfortunately, there is no clue as to the nature of these factors. Experiments in monkeys and sheep have demonstrated that the placenta is capable of compensatory growth. In the rhesus monkey there are usually two placental discs: a primary disc and a smaller, secondary disc. At mid gestation ligation of the fetal blood vessels supplying the secondary disc has shown that the secondary disc undergoes the same changes observed in the whole placenta after fetectomy and that the primary disc increases in weight and DNA content. As alluded to earlier, Alexander (1, 2) attempted to stunt placental growth in sheep by removing caruncles from the nonpregnant uterus. A reduction in the number of caruncles had the expected result of reducing the number of placental cotyledons. In several ewes the reduction in cotyledonary number was compensated for by an increase in cotyledonary weight, so that the aggregate weight of the cotyledons (placental weight) was approximately normal. In some ewes the compensatory growth of the cotyledons in response to carunculectomy was only partial or absent, in which case placental weight was abnormally small.

Placental growth may also depend in part on antigenic differences between mother and fetus. The hemochorial placentas of mouse fetuses that are genetically dissimilar from the mother grow approximately 25% larger than the placentas of fetuses whose parents are from the same genetic strain (4).

REFERENCES

1. Alexander, G. (1964). *Studies on the placenta of the sheep (Ovis aries L.). Effect of surgical reduction in the number of caruncles.* Journal of Reproduction and Fertility **7**, 307–322.
2. Alexander, G. (1974). *Birth weight of lambs: influences and consequences. In* "Size at Birth," Ciba Foundation Symposium 27, pp 215–239, Elsevier-Excerpta Medica-North Holland, Amsterdam.
3. Baur, R. (1977). "Morphometry of the Placental Exchange Area. Advances in Anatomy Embryology and Cell Biology," Springer-Verlag, Berlin.
4. Beer, A.E., Billingham, R.E. and Scott, J.R. (1975). *Immunogenetic aspects of implantation, placentation and fetoplacental growth rates.* Biology of Reproduction **12**, 176–189.
5. Behrman, R.E., Seeds, A.E. Jr., Battaglia, F.C., Hellegers, A.E. and Bruns, P.D. (1964). *The normal changes in mass and water content in fetal rhesus monkey and placenta throughout gestation.* Journal of Pediatrics **65**, 38–44.
6. Carmichael, L. *The relationship of gestation-duration and birth weight in primates. In* "Morphology, Embryology, Functional Anatomy" pp 55–58.
7. Carter, A.M. (1975). *Placental circulation. In* "Comparative Placentation. Essays in Structure and Function," (D.H. Steven, ed.), pp 108–156, Academic Press, New York.
8. Cheek, D.B. (1968). "Human Growth," Lea and Febiger, Philadelphia.
9. Dunn, P.M. (1981). *Variations in fetal growth: Some causes and effects. In* "Fetal Growth Retardation" (F.A. Van Assche and W.B. Robertson, eds.), pp 79–89, Churchill Livingstone, Edinburgh.
9a. Eastman, N.J. and Hellman, L.M. (1966). "Williams Obstetrics," 13th edition. Appleton-Century Crofts, New York.
10. Etienne, M. and Henry, Y. (1973). *Influence d l'apport energetique sur l'utilisation digestive et metabolique des nutriments, et les performances de reproduction chez la truie gestante nullipare.* Annals Zootechnologique **22**, 311–326.
11. Flexner, L.B. and Gellhorn, A. (1942). *The comparative physiology of placental transfer.* American Journal of Obstetrics and Gynecology **43**, 965–974.
12. Freese, V.E. (1972). *Vascular relations of placental exchange areas in primates and man. In* "Respiratory Gas Exchange and Blood Flow in the Placenta" (L.D. Longo and H. Bartels, eds.), pp 31–54, DHEW Publication (NIH) 73–361, Washington, D.C.
13. Friess, A.E., Sinowatz, F., Skolek-Winnisch, R. and Trautner, W. (1980). *The placenta*

of the pig. I. Finestructural changes of the placental barrier during pregnancy. Anatomic Embryology **158**, 179–191.

14. Gehr, P., Sehovic, S., Burri, P.H., Glaassen, H. and Weibel, E.R. (1980). *The lung of shrews: Morphometric estimation of diffusion capacity.* Respiration Physiology **40**, 33–47.

15. Grosser, O. (1909). "Vergleichende Anatomie und Entwicklungsgeschichte der Eihaute und der Placenta," Braumuller, Vienna.

16. Harding, P.G.R. (1970). *Chronic placental insufficiency.* American Journal of Obstetrics and Gynecology **106**, 857.

17. Hofman, M.A. (1983). *Evolution of brain size in neonatal and adult placental mammals: a theoretical approach.* Journal of Theoretical Biology **105**, 317–332.

18. Huggett, A.St.G. and Widdas, W.F. (1951). *The relationship between mammalian foetal weight and conception age.* Journal of Physiology **114**, 306–317.

19. Hugonnaud, C., Gehr, P., Weibel, E.R. and Burri, P.H. (1977). *Adaptation of the growing lung to increased oxygen consumption. II. Morphometric analysis.* Respiration Physiology **29**, 1–10.

20. Koong, L.J., Garrett, W.N. and Rattray, P.V. (1975). *A description of the dynamics of fetal growth in sheep.* Journal of Animal Science **41**, 1065–1068.

21. Kulhanek, J.F., Meschia, G., Makowski, E.L. and Battaglia, F.C. (1974). *Changes in DNA content and urea permeability of the sheep placenta.* American Journal of Physiology **226**, 1257–1263.

22. Lanman, J.T., Mitsudo, S.M., Brinson, A.O. and Thau, R.B. (1975). *Fetectomy in monkeys (Macaca mulatta): Retention of the placenta past normal term.* Biology of Reproduction **12**, 522–525.

23. Leitch, I., Hytten, F.E. and Billewicz, W.Z. (1959). *The maternal and neonatal weights of some mammals.* Proceedings of the Zoological Society, London **133**, 11–28.

24. Mossman, H.W. (1926). *The rabbit placenta and the problem of placental transmission.* American Journal of Anatomy **37**, 433–497.

25. Panigel, M. and Myers, R.E. (1971). *L'effet de la foetectomie et celui de la ligature des vaisseaux foetaux interplacentaires sur l'ultrastructure des villosites placentaires chez Macaca mulatta.* C.R. Academie Sciences Serie D (Paris) **272**, 315–318.

26. Ramsey, E.M. (1973). *Placental vasculature and circulation. In* "Handbook of Physiology. Endocrinology," (R.O. Greep and E.B. Astwood, eds.), Volume II, Section 7, Part 2, Chapter 47, pp 323–337, American Physiologic Society, Bethesda, Maryland.

27. Rattray, P.V., Garret, W.M., East, N.E. and Hinman, N. (1974). *Growth, development and composition of the ovine conceptus and mammary gland during pregnancy.* Journal of Animal Science **38**, 613–629.

28. Sacher, G.A. and Staffeldt, E.F. (1974). *Relation of gestation time to brain weight for placental mammals: Implications for the theory of vertebrate growth.* American Naturalist **198**, 593–615.

29. Silver, M., Steven, D.H. and Comline, R.S. (1973). *Placental exchange and morphology in ruminants and the mare. In* "Foetal and Neonatal Physiology" (K.S. Comline, K.W. Cross, G.S. Dawes and P.W. Nathanielzs, eds.), Proceedings of the Sir Joseph Barcroft Centenary Symposium, pp 245–271, Cambridge University Press, Cambridge.

30. Sparks, J.W., Girard, J.R. and Battaglia, F.C. (1980). *An estimate of the caloric requirements of the human fetus.* Biology of the Neonate **38**, 113–119.

31. Sparks, J.W., Girard, J.R., Callikan, S. and Battaglia, F.C. (1985) *Growth of fetal guinea pig: Physical and chemical characteristics.* American Journal of Physiology **248**, E132–E139.

32. Steven, D.H. (1975). *Anatomy of the placental barrier. In* "Comparative Placentation. Essays in Structure and Function," (D.H. Steven, ed.), pp 25–56, Academic Press, New York.

33. Tsutsumi, Y. (1962). Journal of Agriculture, Hokkaido (imp.) University **52,** 372–482.

34. Tyndale-Biscoe, H. (1973). "Life of Marsupials," Edward Arnold (Publishers) Limited, London.

35. Widdowson, E.M. (1974). *Changes in body proportion and composition during growth. In* "Scientific Foundations of Paediatrics" (J.A. Davis and J. Dobbing, eds.), pp 44–55, W.B. Saunders Company, Philadelphia.

36. Ziegler, E.E., O'Donnell, A.M., Nelson, S.E. and Fomon, S.J. (1979). *Body composition of the reference fetus.* Growth **40,** 329–341.

2

Transplacental Diffusion: Basic Concepts

A SIMPLE MODEL

The placenta can be considered an organ designed for the transfer of heat and matter between two streams (maternal and fetal placental blood flows). As such, it is part of a class of devices, commonly known as exchangers, of which there are several other examples in biology (e.g., lungs and gills) and in engineering (e.g., heat exchangers and dialyzers).

What kind of measurements and calculations are needed to understand how the placental exchanger works and to evaluate its performance? The answer to this question is complex but can be clarified by a stepwise approach. The first step is to acquire some basic concepts from the study of a simple exchanger operating under steady-state conditions. The quantities that we will be dealing with, their units of measurements, and symbols are listed in Table 2-1.

Imagine an exchanger (Figure 2-1) consisting of a membrane of uniform composition and thickness that separates two vigorously stirred compartments (compartments I and II). An aqueous solution flows at a constant rate (F for compartment I and f for compartment II) through each of the compartments. Assume further that a solute x is entering at a constant arterial concentration into each compartment (A_x and a_x) and diffusing at constant rate from compartment II to compartment I. The solute cannot

28

Table 2-1

Explanation of Symbols and Units for Model in Figure 2-1

Symbol	Definition	Unit
F	Flow of solution through compartment I	ml/min
f	Flow of solution through compartment II	ml/min
A_x	Arterial concentration of solute x, entering compartment I	mg/ml
V_x	Venous concentration of solute x, exiting compartment I	mg/ml
a_x	Arterial concentration of solute x, entering compartment II	mg/ml
v_x	Venous concentration of solute x, exiting compartment II	mg/ml
R_x	Net rate of transfer of solute x from II to I	mg/min
P_x	Permeability to solute x	ml/min

be metabolized or produced by the exchanger, and it is electrically neutral and exists in each solution in the free form only (inert solute). Its concentration in each part of the system is constant with time. The principle of conservation of matter tells us that the rate of entry of solute x in one of the compartments must equal its rate of exit from that compartment. Therefore for compartment I (using the symbols in Table 2-1),

$$A_x F + R_x = V_x F \tag{2-1}$$

and for compartment II

$$a_x f = R_x + v_x f \tag{2-2}$$

By rearrangement of these equations

$$R_x = F(V_x - A_x) = f(a_x - v_x) \tag{2-3}$$

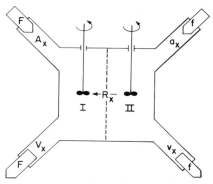

Figure 2-1:   Double pool, venous equilibrator model of placental exchange. The meaning of each symbol is explained in Table 2-1.

(In physiology, the principle stating that under steady-state conditions the product of flow times arteriovenous difference equals net uptake by an organ or a compartment is known as the Fick principle.) Equation 2-3 is valid for any exchanger, no matter how complex, as long as the diffusing molecule is not metabolized or produced within the exchanger and the system is in a steady state.

Our next step is to establish the quantitative relationship of transfer rate of $x(R_x)$ to the flow rates (F and f) at which the two solutions perfuse compartments I and II, and the permeability (P_x) of the membrane. We begin by considering permeability.

According to Fick's law of diffusion (not to be confused with the Fick principle), the rate of transfer of solute x from compartment II to I is related to the concentration difference between the two compartments, and to the area and thickness of the membrane by the equation

$$R_x = D_x \frac{\text{area}}{\text{thickness}} \text{ (concentration difference)} \tag{2-4}$$

where D_x is the diffusion coefficient of the membrane for substance x. For any given membrane and temperature, $D_x(\text{area}/\text{thickness})$ is a constant. We call this constant "permeability of the exchanger for substance x" (symbol P_x). Therefore,

$$R_x = P_x(\text{concentration difference}) \tag{2-5}$$

Note that permeability is the proportionality coefficient between transfer rate and the concentration difference across the membrane. The units of measurement of P are milliliters per minute.

In the simple model of Figure 2-1, the concentrations of x to which the membrane is exposed are the venous concentrations of the exchanger. This is so because the vigorous stirring is assumed to create a solution of uniform composition within each compartment. Therefore,

$$R_x = P_x(v_x - V_x) \tag{2-6}$$

To show how the rates of perfusion of the two solutions influence transfer, we make use again of the Fick principle and rearrange Equation 2-3 to express each venous concentration as a function of the flow, the transfer rate and arterial concentration:

$$v_x = a_x - \frac{R_x}{f} \tag{2-7}$$

and

$$V_x = A_x + \frac{R_x}{F} \tag{2-8}$$

We then use Equations 2-7 and 2-8 to eliminate v_x and V_x from Equation 2-6, with the result

$$R_x = \frac{a_x - A_x}{1/P + 1/F + 1/f} \tag{2-9}$$

Equation 2-9 shows how the transplacental diffusion rate is related to arterial concentrations, permeability, and flows.

PLACENTAL CLEARANCE: DEFINITION AND PROPERTIES

The absolute value of the transfer rate : arterial concentration difference ratio has been termed by us (10, 11) the *placental clearance* (C). For the model of Figure 2-1,

$$C_x = \frac{1}{1/P + 1/F + 1/f} \tag{2-10}$$

It is important to understand why we sometimes focus attention on clearance rather than transfer rate in placental physiology. The direction and magnitude of the transfer rate depend upon arterial concentrations, which in many cases can be set arbitrarily at any value by the experimenter and without changing the properties of the exchanger. Therefore placental transfer rate is not a satisfactory index of placental function. To the contrary, clearance depends exclusively on the properties of the exchanger. This is, of course, the same reason why we consider renal clearances to be valid indices of renal function, whereas rates of urinary excretion are not.

Implicit in Equation 2-10 are three important concepts. The first is that clearance would be zero if either permeability or one of the two flows were zero. This supports the intuition that a permeable membrane and perfusion of the membrane on both sides are essential elements for any steady transfer to occur. The second concept is that the clearance of different inert solutes varies between two limits: (a) permeability limited clearance and (b) flow-limited clearance. Assume a situation in which F and f are much higher than P_x (flows and permeability are expressed in the same units of milliliters per minute and are thus directly comparable). In this situation, the numerical value of $(1/F + 1/f)$ would be negligible in comparison to $1/P_x$ and therefore,

$$C_x = P_x \tag{2-11}$$

In other words, if permeability is much less than flows, clearance is virtually equal to, and limited by, membrane permeability. Conversely, assume a situation in which permeability is much higher than flows. In this case, $1/P_x$ is negligible in comparison $(1/F + 1/f)$ and the clearance is limited by the rate of perfusion of the exchanger, according to the equation

$$C_x = \frac{1}{1/F + 1/f} = \frac{F \times f}{F + f} \qquad (2\text{-}12)$$

The third concept is that, for a given membrane and sets of flow, the flow-limited clearance is the maximum clearance of the exchanger. That is, if we tested the exchanger with a series of inert solutes having different permeability coefficients in the membrane (D_x), we would observe that as the permeability coefficient D_x increases toward large values, there is an increase of the clearance toward the asymtotic maximum represented by the flow-limited clearance.

PLACENTAL EFFECTIVENESS (Transfer Index)

We have selected the double pool model of Figure 2-1 for the introduction of basic concepts because in this model the relationship of clearance to flows and permeability can be defined by a simple equation (Equation 2-10). However, equations that apply to other models are more complex. For this reason, several investigators have preferred to use graphic representations of these relationships. Such representations can assume many different forms because they attempt to illustrate by means of two-dimensional graphs the dependence of clearance on three independent variables. Some investigators have used plots which illustrate the dependence of clearance : flow ratios on permeability : flow and flow : flow ratios. The clearance : flow ratio has been named *effectiveness* by Moll and Kastendieck (13) and *transfer index* by Faber (4, 5). Note the following equalities:

$$\frac{C_x}{F} = \frac{V_x - A_x}{a_x - A_x} \qquad (2\text{-}13)$$

and

$$\frac{C_x}{f} = \frac{a_x - v_x}{a_x - A_x} \qquad (2\text{-}14)$$

Therefore, the effectiveness (transfer index) of an exchanger is nothing more than the arteriovenous difference across one of the two circulations "normalized" for the artery to artery concentration difference between the two circulations.

VENOUS EQUILIBRATORS AND COUNTERCURRENT EXCHANGERS

The next step in our analysis is to establish the importance of flow patterns within an exchanger in determining its performance. The exchanger which we have studied thus far (Figure 2-1) is a "venous equilibrator." In this type of exchanger and under conditions of flow-limited clearance, the venous concentration in the donor stream is virtually equal to the venous concentration in the recipient stream. Another type of venous equilibrator is the concurrent exchanger which consists of a membrane separating two streams running in the same direction (Figure 2-2).

CONCURRENT

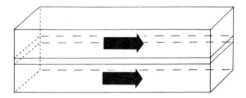

COUNTERCURRENT

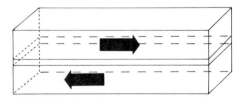

MULTICAPILLARY

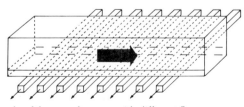

Figure 2-2: Example of three exchangers with different flow arrangements. The multicapillary exchanger has been considered by some workers to be a model of the human placenta, but the physiologic evidence to support this model is lacking (9).

The details of the relationship among clearance, permeability, and flows vary among the different types of venous equilibrators. For example, in the concurrent exchanger the relationship is as follows:

$$C_x = \frac{F \times f}{F + f}\left\{1 - \exp\left[-P_x\left(\frac{1}{F} + \frac{1}{f}\right)\right]\right\} \qquad (2\text{-}15)$$

where exp is the base of the natural log. However, in every venous equilibrator, the relationship of flow-limited clearance to flows is as shown by Equation 2-12.

Imagine now that the concurrent exchanger were to be transformed into a countercurrent exchanger by reversing the direction of one of the two flows (Figure 2-2). This transformation creates a more efficient system of exchange because the venous output of one stream tends to equilibrate with the arterial input of the other stream. The equation relating clearance to permeability and flows in a countercurrent exchanger is complex. Therefore, it is more convenient to illustrate the properties of the counter-current exchanger graphically. In a graph of effectiveness versus per-meability : flow ratio (Figure 2-3) with the two flows assumed to be equal, we see that at low permeability values the countercurrent and concurrent exchangers have approximately the same level of performance. However, as the transfer rate becomes flow limited (i.e., as the permeability : flow ratio increases to very large values), the countercurrent exchanger has a definite advantage. If the flow-limited effectiveness is plotted against the maternal : fetal flow ratio (Figure 2-4), it can be seen that the maximum

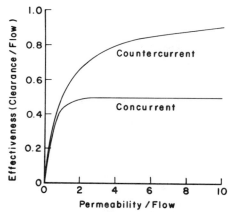

Figure 2-3: Relation of effectiveness to the permeability : flow ratio exchangers with flow ratio = 1. In both the countercurrent and concurrent models of placental exchange, effectiveness tends toward a flow-limited maximum as permeability increases in relationship to perfusion rate.

advantage of the countercurrent exchanger is at flow ratios that are close to 1.

It is important to realize that the greater effectiveness of a placenta that behaves like a countercurrent exchanger can be exploited physiologically in two radically different ways (the "fetal advantage" and the "maternal advantage") which are illustrated by the models in Figure 2-5. Consider first a model (panel I) in which maternal and fetal placental blood flows are arranged to form a concurrent exchanger for the purpose of transferring substance x from mother to fetus at the rate of 50 μmol/min. The transfer is by passive diffusion and is flow limited. With a maternal : fetal flow ratio of 2, a maternal arterial concentration of 100 μM is associated with umbilical arterial and venous concentrations of 25 and 75 μM, respectively. Next, we make the exchanger more effective by reversing the direction of maternal blood flow while its magnitude is kept constant. The result of this maneuver is shown in the panel II of Figure 2-5. The fetus can now draw the same amount of substance x from the mother, but it does so with a concentration of x in fetal blood which is much higher than it was with the concurrent arrangement. To obtain this result, we left the rate of maternal perfusion unchanged. Thus, the fetus is the exclusive beneficiary of the switch from the concurrent to the countercurrent mode of exchange (fetal advantage). Suppose, however, that we were not interested in increasing the concentration of substance x in fetal blood and wanted to make the mother the exclusive beneficiary of the countercurrent arrangement. In this case maternal placental blood flow is reduced

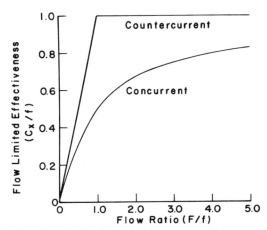

Figure 2-4: The flow-limited effectiveness of a venous equilibrator (represented in this case by a concurrent exchanger) is generally less than the effectiveness of a countercurrent exchanger. The largest difference in effectiveness occurs at a flow ratio of 1.0.

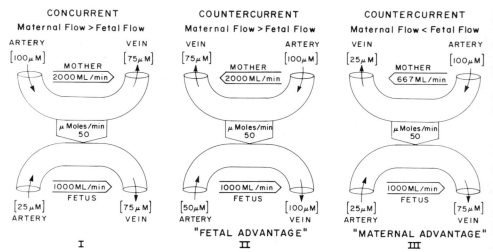

Figure 2-5: The physiologic advantage of a placenta with countercurrent perfusion can be used to minimize the maternal–fetal arterial concentration differences of diffusing molecules (fetal advantage) or to reduce maternal placental blood flow well below the level required by a less effective placenta (maternal advantage).

until the concentration of substance x in fetal blood is the same as it was with the concurrent arrangement. As demonstrated in panel III of Figure 2-5, the maternal advantage would be substantial in this case, for the mother could now provide the same fetal environment and rate of placental transfer with a placental blood flow which is only one-third of the rate required by a venous equilibrator. Among mammals one can find examples of placentas which are venous equilibrators (e.g., sheep), placentas which are similar to countercurrent exchangers with ''fetal advantage'' (e.g., horse), and placentas which are similar to countercurrent exchangers with ''maternal advantage'' (e.g., guinea pig). This important aspect of comparative physiology is further discussed in Chapters 6 and 8.

APPLICATION OF THE CONCEPT OF FLOW-LIMITED CLEARANCE TO COMPLEX EXCHANGERS

The exchangers which we have discussed thus far differ substantially in their geometry and/or performance, but they all share the property of having a maximum flow-limited clearance at high levels of permeability. Since it may seem intuitive that this is a general property of exchangers, it is important to realize that there are some exchangers in which maximum

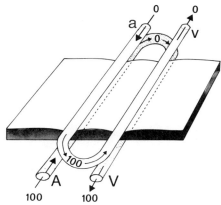

Figure 2-6: Hypothetical double countercurrent exchanger formed by a maternal and a fetal capillary loop. Maternal blood enters at point A carrying a highly diffusible substance with concentration 100 and runs in the opposite direction to fetal blood entering at point a with concentration 0. At the end of arterial branches of the two loops, fetal concentration is 100 and maternal concentration is 0. The two streams run countercurrent again in the venous branches of the loops (V, v), and consequently, maternal concentration increases to 100 and fetal concentration returns to 0. The result is no net transfer of highly diffusible substance from mother to fetus (9).

clearance does not occur when the permeability is at its maximum (5, 15). For example, consider the exchanger depicted in Figure 2-6. A maternal and a fetal capillary loop face each other across a membrane to form what has been called a "double countercurrent exchanger" (5). If we assume that the two loops carry equal flows, it can be shown the maximum transfer rate is obtained when the permeability of the tissues interposed between maternal and fetal blood is equal to flow (5). Paradoxically, as the permeability tends to infinity, the net rate of transfer between the two circulations tends to zero as shown in Figure 2-6. Because of such theoretical considerations, an important task in placental physiology has been to determine whether the concept of flow-limited maximum clearance is applicable to the placenta of a given species by the collection of appropriate experimental data.

PLACENTAL TRANSFER OF INERT MOLECULES

The theoretical discussion of exchangers delineates the information which is needed in order to characterize the placenta of a particular species as the organ of exchange between mother and fetus: measurements of maternal and fetal placental blood flows, transplacental diffusion rates of

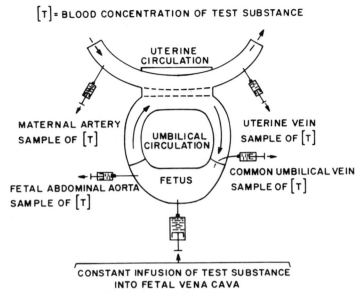

$[T]$ = BLOOD CONCENTRATION OF TEST SUBSTANCE

Figure 2-7: Scheme of experimental design for studying transplacental diffusion *in vivo* under steady-state conditions and for the simultaneous measurement of uterine and umbilical blood flows (12).

various test molecules; and their concentrations in the arteries and veins of both placental vascular beds, umbilical and uterine.

In response to the specific information required for such an analysis, the following experimental preparation was developed for sheep (10, 11). Catheters to be used for blood sampling are inserted in a maternal artery, a large uterine vein, one fetal femoral artery (which carries blood of the same composition as that perfusing the umbilical artery), and the umbilical vein. A fifth catheter is placed in a fetal femoral vein and connected to an infusion pump in which a solution of one or more test substances is infused at a constant rate (Figure 2-7). Consider first what happens when the test substance is antipyrine, a relatively inert substance that diffuses rapidly in all body compartments. The infusion pump containing the antipyrine solution is started at time zero. Then, sets of blood samples are withdrawn simultaneously from the maternal artery, the uterine vein, the fetal femoral artery, and the umbilical vein. These samples are analyzed for antipyrine concentration, and the results of the analysis are plotted versus time. If the animal preparation is stable, the data we obtain are as depicted in Figure 2-8. Observe that antipyrine concentration rises rapidly in fetal blood during the first 40 min of the infusion. This rise establishes a

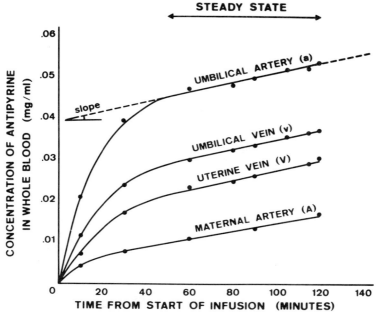

STEADY STATE

Figure 2-8: Concentrations of antipyrine in fetal and maternal blood during the continuous infusion of antipyrine in the femoral vein of a fetal lamb. Infusion rate = 10 mg/min; fetal weight = 3750 g; fetal body water = 3000 ml (8).

transplacental concentration gradient that promotes diffusion of the test substance from fetus to mother and slows down its accumulation in the fetal body. The end result is the automatic attainment of a steady state in which the arteriovenous concentration differences across the umbilical and uterine circulations are constant and the rise of antipyrine concentration in fetal blood is reduced to a minimum. During this steady state we can use the data to obtain some important information, which is summarized in Table 2-2.

The critical calculation is that of the transplacental diffusion rate of antipyrine. When an inert substance is infused into the fetal circulation, it either accumulates in the fetal body or escapes (by definition, if it is inert, it is not metabolized). The rate of accumulation can be estimated from the slope of the blood concentration and its distribution volume within fetal body water. In the numerical example of Figure 2-8 and Table 2-2, the slope is 0.000118 mg/ml/min and the antipyrine volume of distribution is equal to total body water (3000 ml). Therefore, antipyrine accumulation rate in the fetus is the product of these two numbers, or 0.35 mg/min. It

Table 2-2

Calculations Based on the Data of Figure 2-8

Fetal body water = 3000 ml
Antipyrine infusion rate = 10 mg/min
Accumulation rate of antipyrine in the fetus = 0.000118 ×
    3000 = 0.35 mg/min
Transplacental diffusion rate of antipyrine = 10 − 0.35 =
    9.65 mg/min
$a - v$ = 0.0163 mg/ml
Umbilical blood flow = 9.65/0.0163 = 592 ml/min
$V - A$ = 0.0138 mg/ml
Uterine blood flow = 9.65/0.0138 = 699 ml/min
Antipyrine clearance = 9.65/0.0375 = 257 ml/min

follows that if the infusion rate is 10.00 mg/min and the accumulation rate is 0.35 mg/min, then the rate of escape must be 10.00 − 0.35 = 9.65 mg/min. In the numerical example of Table 2-2, we have assumed that the placenta is the only route of escape for antipyrine from fetus to mother. In which case

Transplacental diffusion rate = infusion rate − escape rate

A more refined calculation would include a consideration that some antipyrine can escape the fetal body via the fetal kidneys and that some metabolism of the drug takes place. However, for antipyrine it has been shown that these are small corrections. The important concept is that infusion of an inert substance at a constant rate into the fetal circulation establishes a known and constant rate of diffusion of the test substance across the placenta while the fetus is *in utero* and under normal physiologic conditions. Once the transplacental diffusion rate is known, several calculations derive from that. These include the following.

The placental clearance of antipyrine is calculated as the ratio of transplacental diffusion rate over the concentration difference between umbilical arterial blood and maternal arterial blood. Umbilical blood flow is calculated by applying the same reasoning used in the study of the elementary exchangers (Fick principle). Since each milliliter of umbilical blood delivers 0.0163 mg of antipyrine to the placenta, the amount of umbilical blood needed to deliver 9.65 mg/min must be 9.65/0.0163 = 592 ml/min. Similarly, we apply the same principle to the uptake of antipyrine by the uterine circulation and calculate the uterine blood flow to be 699 ml/min.

The experimental design which we have described creates a situation in which the placenta performs the function of transferring from fetus to mother an inert substance at a constant rate and under steady-state conditions. The next step is to analyze this performance. First, to evaluate the performance of the placenta as an exchanger, we need to know whether the concept of a flow-limited maximum clearance is applicable to the placenta despite its complexity. If this proves to be the case, we need to measure maternal and fetal placental blood flows in order to compare flow-limited clearance with flows. The comparison of flow-limited placental clearance with total uterine and umbilical flows would not be adequate because part of the total uterine flow does not go through the placenta but perfuses the myometrium.

In studying the theory of elementary exchangers, we have seen that for a given set of flows the flow-limited clearance is also the maximal clearance, which is common to all molecules to which the membrane is highly permeable. This property suggests the approach by which we can ascertain whether the placenta has a measurable flow-limited clearance. Again, this approach is analogous to that originally used to define GFR in the kidney. We infuse simultaneously into the fetal circulation a mixture of substances that diffuse rapidly across the placenta and have radically different physicochemical properties. If these substances have the same placental clearance, we may conclude that their clearance is a maximum, that is, their differing permeabilities are not determinants of the transfer and that the placenta has indeed a measurable flow-limited clearance. Table 2-3 shows a comparison of placental clearances of tritiated water, antipyrine, and ethanol in sheep. It is apparent that the clearances of these three substances are virtually the same despite marked differences in physicochemical properties. Therefore, the clearance of these molecules is indeed a measure of the placental flow-limited clearance of inert molecules.

It has been possible to measure myoendometrial, endometrial and cotyledonary blood flows in sheep by means of the microsphere technique (see

Table 2-3

A Comparison of Physico-Chemical Properties of ^3H_2O, Antipyrine and Ethanol, and Their Placental Clearances

	^3H_2O	Ethanol	Antipyrine	Reference
Molecular weight	19	46	188	
Partition coefficient, ether/water	0.003	0.26	0.073	2
Permeability, red cells (cm/sec) $\times 10^{-5}$	915	8.8	—	14
Reflection coefficient, gall bladder	0.000	0.050	0.370	17
Placental clearance ratio, sheep				
(^3H_2O ratio = 1)	1.0	1.09	1.02	3, 10

Chapter 8). In late gestation but prior to the contractions of labor, myometrial blood flow is a small fraction (approximately 3%) of uterine blood flow (7). Most of the uterine blood flow is to the placental cotyledons (approximately 84%) and the endometrium (approximately 13%). Since the endometrial circulation could participate in the maternal-fetal exchange of highly diffusible molecules, we conclude that in late gestation the uterine and umbilical blood flows closely represent the two blood flows of the placental exchanger.

Given the above information, let us reconsider the data in Figure 2-8 and Table 2-2. We notice first that the antipyrine clearance is much less than the smaller of the two flows (257 versus 592 ml/min). This demonstrates that the level of performance of the ovine placenta is much below that of a countercurrent exchanger. In an ideal countercurrent exchanger, flow-limited clearance is equal to the lesser of the two flows. Is the level of performance equal to that of a venous equilibrator? We have seen that in an ideal venous equilibrator, the flow-limited clearance is equal to the product of the flows divided by their sum (Equation 2-12). Therefore, in the example of Table 2-2, placental exchange could be said to be equal to that of a venous equilibrator if the antipyrine clearance were $(699 \times 592)/(699 + 592) = 320$ ml/min. In fact, the antipyrine clearance is 257 ml/min, which is 20% less than the calculated value. This discrepancy, which has been observed in numerous experiments, indicates that in sheep the uterine and umbilical blood flows form an exchanger which is somewhat less effective than an ideal venous equilibrator. Several factors are likely to contribute to this ineffectiveness. The myometrial "shunt" is one factor; another factor is uneven placental perfusion. The placenta is made up of numerous exchange units, each having somewhat different maternal : fetal blood flow ratios. Uneven perfusion decreases the effectiveness of the whole exchanger. A third factor is the arrangement of maternal and fetal arterioles which run within the placental cotyledon in close proximity to vascular channels that carry blood from the exchange area. Because of this arrangement, molecules can diffuse directly from artery to vein in the donor stream and from vein to artery in the recipient stream, thus creating "diffusional shunts."

In a placenta that functions as a venous equilibrator, the rate at which a substance is transferred between the uterine and umbilical circulation is a nonlinear function of uterine blood flow. (Figure 2-4 presents the theoretical relationship of flow-limited effectiveness to flow ratio in a concurrent exchanger.) The experimental verification of this important concept is shown in Figure 2-9. Placental ethanol clearance was measured in six sheep at different levels of uterine blood flow (16). In each animal norepinephrine infusion, maternal hemorrhage, or occlusion of the terminal

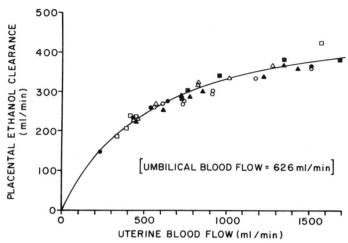

Figure 2-9: Relationship of ethanol clearance to uterine blood flow at constant umbilical blood flow of 626 ml/min. Each animal is represented by a separate symbol. Curve was drawn according to Equation 2-16 in text (16).

aorta were used to reduce uterine blood flow below normal. Umbilical flow did not covary with uterine flow, but varied at random within relatively narrow limits around a mean of 626 ml/min. Multiple regression analysis of clearance versus uterine and umbilical flows showed the ethanol clearance (C_E) to be a function of uterine (F) and umbilical (f) flows according to the equation

$$C_E = \frac{1}{1/0.911F + 1/0.831f} \tag{2-16}$$

Note that the numerical coefficients in this equation (0.911 and 0.831) are less than 1 and represent a measure of the combined effects of shunts and uneven perfusion in lowering the effectiveness of the exchange between the uterine and the umbilical circulations. In Figure 2-9 the curve drawn through the experimental points is the graphic expression of Equation 2-16 for a constant umbilical flow of 626 ml/min. Implicit in this curvilinear relation is the concept of an optimal uterine:umbilical blood flow ratio. On the one hand, if uterine blood flow is much less than umbilical blood flow, placental transfer can be inadequate. On the other hand, if uterine blood flow is much higher than umbilical blood flow, the exchange system is used inefficiently in that a large increment of maternal perfusion, presumably at the expense of maternal cardiac workload, is associated with a small increment in the rate of transfer. The problem of optimizing the uterine : umbilical blood flow ratio can be put in the following terms. Given a fixed amount of blood that can be used to perfuse either the maternal or fetal surface of the placental membrane or both, what should the relative perfusion of each side be to attain a maximum clearance of inert molecules? Intuitively, it appears that maximum clearance will occur when each side receives equal blood flows. Both experimental and theoretical evidence (Figure 2-10) confirm this supposition by showing that the clearance : (uterine flow + umbilical flow) ratio is maximal when the uterine flow : umbilical flow ratio is approximately 1.0. We cannot assume, however, that a uterine flow : umbilical flow ratio which is optimal for the transfer of inert molecules will also be optimal for the placental transfer of biologically active molecules, such as oxygen. In the case of oxygen transfer other important factors, that is, oxygen capacity and oxygen affinity of maternal and fetal blood as well as the oxygen consumption rate of the placenta, must be taken into consideration.

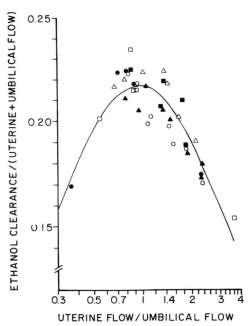

Figure 2-10: Given a certain amount of total placental perfusion (uterine + umbilical blood flow), there is maximum clearance when the uterine : umbilical blood flow ratio is approximately 1.0. Each animal is represented by a separate symbol (16).

PLACENTAL PERMEABILITY

The properties of the placenta that promote the exchange of molecules between mother and fetus are sometimes referred to as "placental permeability." This broad concept of permeability includes many different mechanisms (e.g., passive diffusion and active transfer) and different factors (e.g., placental perfusion rate and placental metabolic activity). For these reasons, it is unsuited for a quantitative analysis of transplacental exchange. A more precise definition of permeability has been used in studying the passive diffusion of metabolically inert molecules across the placental barrier (1, 6). In these studies, placental permeability was defined as the proportionality coefficient relating the net rate of transplacental diffusion to the mean concentration difference between maternal and fetal plasma water. This definition conforms to the concept of permeability in Fick's law of diffusion (Equation 2-5). In respiratory physiology a coefficient of analogous meaning is called *diffusing capacity*. Thus, the expressions *placental diffusing capacity* and *placental permeability* have been used interchangeably.

For inert molecules whose placental clearance is much smaller than the blood flow-limited clearance, clearance and permeability are virtually identical, i.e., the clearance is permeability limited (Equation 2-11). This is because the arteriovenous concentration differences of the diffusing substance are quite small. As a consequence, the maternal-fetal arterial concentration difference is nearly equal to the mean concentration difference across the placental barrier.

However, in many instances the placental clearance of a substance can be limited in part by the rate of placental perfusion and in part by placental permeability. When this occurs, placental clearance is appreciably less than placental permeability and the calculation of permeability becomes more difficult.

The permeability (diffusing capacity) of the sheep placenta to urea has been calculated by measuring the placental clearances of antipyrine and urea simultaneously (6). In this calculation two basic assumptions were made: (a) that the antipyrine clearance represents the flow-limited clearance of inert molecules and (b) that the sheep placenta is a concurrent exchanger. In a concurrent exchanger (see Equation 2-15),

$$C_u = C_{max}(1 - e^{-P_u/C_{max}}) \qquad (2\text{-}17)$$

where C_u, C_{max}, and P_u represent urea clearance, the flow-limited clearance, and urea permeability, respectively. Thus,

$$P_u = C_{max} \ln \frac{C_{max}}{C_{max} - C_u} \qquad (2\text{-}18)$$

To use a numerical example, if C_{max} and C_u are equal to 273 and 66 ml/min, respectively, P_u equals 75.6 ml/min. In the case of urea, the perfusion limitation on clearance is not large. Thus, only a moderate degree of uncertainty is introduced by the assumptions used in the calculations of permeability. For instance, if we were to assume that the model presented in Figure 2-1 represents the sheep placenta more realistically than a concurrent model, we would use a different equation and calculate a larger permeability value:

$$P_u = \frac{C_{max}C_u}{C_{max} - C_u} = \frac{273 \times 66}{273 - 66} = 87.0 \qquad (2\text{-}19)$$

For molecules with higher permeability coefficients than urea, the effect of perfusion limitation is greater and consequently it becomes very difficult to make an exact estimate of permeability. The importance of permeability measurements in establishing the concept of placental functional maturation was discussed in Chapter 1.

Placental Transfer of Inert Molecules in the Guinea Pig

For technical reasons there have been no studies of placental transfer in small mammals under chronic steady-state conditions. However, the performance of the guinea pig placenta in transferring molecules such as nitrous oxide and tritiated water has been studied in artificially perfused preparations (13). As shown in Figure 2-11, which compares data for the

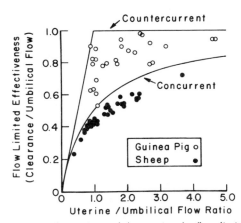

Figure 2-11: Comparison of experimental data testing the flow-limited effectiveness of the guinea pig and sheep placenta. Guinea pig data from Moll and Kastendieck (13); sheep data from Wilkening et al. (16).

sheep and guinea pig placentas, the effectiveness of the guinea pig placenta is substantially higher than that of a venous equilibrator at any level of uterine : umbilical flow ratio, in agreement with histologic studies indicating that the guinea pig placenta simulates a countercurrent exchanger. The data in the guinea pig experiments show a high degree of variability in comparison to the data in sheep, but this has no physiologic significance since it is likely to represent the instability of an artificially perfused preparation in contrast to a chronic *in vivo* preparation. The fundamental observation is that the relationship of placental effectiveness to the uterine : umbilical flow ratio is radically different in the two species.

REFERENCES

1. Battaglia, F.C., Behrman, R.E., Meschia, G., Seeds, A.E. and Bruns, P.D. (1968). *Clearance of inert molecules, Na and Cl ions across the primate placenta.* American Journal of Obstetrics and Gynecology **102,** 1135–1143.
2. Bissonnette, J.M., Cronan, J.Z., Richards, L.L. and Wickham, W.K. (1979). *Placental transfer of water and nonelectrolytes during a simple circulatory passage.* American Journal of Physiology **236,** C47–C52.
3. Bonds, D.R., Anderson, S. and Meschia, G. (1980). *Transplacental diffusion of ethanol under steady state conditions.* Journal of Developmental Physiology **2,** 409–416.
4. Faber, J.J. (1969). *Application of the theory of heat exchangers to the transfer of inert materials in placentas.* Circulation Research **24,** 221–234.
5. Faber, J.J. (1977). *Steady-state methods for the study of placental exchange.* Federation Proceedings **36,** 2640–2646.
6. Kulhanek, J.F., Meschia, G., Makowski, E.L. and Battaglia, F.C. (1974). *Changes in DNA content and urea permeability of the sheep placenta.* American Journal of Physiology **226,** 1257–1263.
7. Makowski, E.L., Meschia, G., Droegemueller, W. and Battaglia, F.C. (1968). *Distribution of uterine blood flow in the pregnant sheep.* American Journal of Obstetrics and Gynecology **101,** 409–412.
8. Meschia, G. (1976). *Physiology of transplacental diffusion. In* "Obstetrics and Gynecology Annual," (R.M. Wynn, ed.), pp 21–38. Appleton-Century-Crofts, New York.
9. Meschia, G. (1983). *Circulation to female reproductive organs. In* "Handbook of Physiology. The Cardiovascular System III," (J.T. Shepherd and F.M. Abboud, eds.), pp 241–269, American Physiologic Society, Bethesda, Maryland.
10. Meschia, G., Battaglia, F.C. and Bruns, P.D. (1967). *Theoretical and experimental study of transplacental diffusion.* Journal of Applied Physiology **22,** 1171–1178.
11. Meschia, G., Cotter, J.R., Makowski, E.L. and Barron, D.H. (1967). *Simultaneous measurement of uterine and umbilical blood flows and oxygen uptakes.* Quarterly Journal of Experimental Physiology **52,** 1–18.
12. Meschia, G., Battaglia, F.C., Hay, W.W. Jr. and Sparks, J.W. (1980). *Utilization of substrates by the ovine placenta in vivo.* Federation Proceedings **39,** 245–249.
13. Moll, W. and Kastendieck, E. (1977). *Transfer of N_2O, CO, and HTO in the artificially perfused guinea pig placenta.* Respiratory Physiology **29,** 283–302.
14. Naccache, P. and Sha'afi, R.I. (1973). *Patterns of nonelectrolyte permeability in human red blood cell membrane.* Journal of General Physiology **62,** 714–736.

15. Rankin, J.H.G. (1972). *The effects of shunted and unevenly distributed blood flows on cross-current exchange in the sheep placenta. In* "Respiratory Gas Exchange and Blood Flow in the Placenta," (L.D. Longo and H. Bartels, eds.), pp 207–226, U.S. DHEW Publication #(NIH) 73–36l.
16. Wilkening, R.B., Anderson, S., Martensson, L. and Meschia, G. (1982). *Placental transfer as a function of uterine blood flow.* American Journal of Physiology **242**, H429–H436.
17. Wright, E.M. and Diamond, J.M. (1969). *Patterns of nonelectrolyte permeability.* Proceedings of the Royal Society of London, Biological Sciences **172**, 227–271.

3

Fetal and Placental Metabolism: Part I. Oxygen and Carbohydrates

CONCEPTS AND TECHNIQUES

Application of the Fick Principle

Measurements of the net fluxes of metabolic substrates between maternal blood and pregnant uterus and between placenta and fetal blood form the basis of our knowledge of placental and fetal metabolism. Several of the measurements rely on the principle of conservation of matter as it applies to the exchange of metabolic substrates between an organ and its circulation (Fick principle). The principle can be stated as follows: in a given time period, the quantity of substrate entering an organ via the arterial blood must be equal to the quantity of substrate being removed from the blood by the organ plus the quantity of substrate leaving in the outflowing venous blood (64). To understand how the Fick principle is applied, let us consider an experiment upon pregnant sheep in which we wish to measure the simultaneous net fluxes of oxygen, glucose, and lactic acid between maternal blood and pregnant uterus and between placenta and fetal blood. A sheep is prepared as described in Chapter 2, i.e., with a fetal venous infusion catheter and catheters for sampling maternal

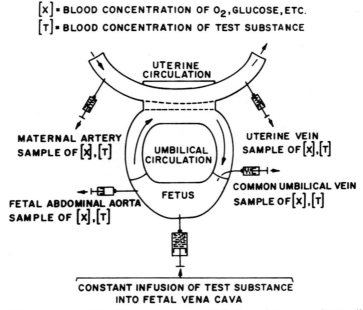

$[x]$ = BLOOD CONCENTRATION OF O$_2$, GLUCOSE, ETC.

$[T]$ = BLOOD CONCENTRATION OF TEST SUBSTANCE

Figure 3-1: Diagram of the sites of sampling and infusion catheters in a chronically catheterized sheep for studies of net umbilical and uterine oxygen and glucose fluxes. This is the same basic design presented in Chapter 2, Figure 2-7 (57).

arterial, uterine venous, umbilical arterial, and venous blood (Figure 3-1). After recovery from surgery, a test molecule (e.g., antipyrine or tritiated water) is infused into the fetus at a constant rate for the purpose of simultaneously measuring uterine and umbilical blood flows. In the steady state, four sets of samples are drawn from the maternal artery, the uterine vein, the fetal artery, and the umbilical vein and are analyzed for whole blood oxygen, glucose, and lactate concentrations. The data on blood flow and metabolic substrate concentrations are then used to calculate the net fluxes of oxygen, glucose, and lactate between the uterine circulation and the pregnant uterus and between the placenta and the umbilical circulation. The rates of oxygen and glucose utilization and of lactate production by the uteroplacental mass are then calculated from the uterine and umbilical fluxes. Table 3-1 gives a numerical example of such calculations. Although the Fick principle is conceptually straightforward, its practical application can give inaccurate results if a number of conditions are not satisfied.

Measurements of concentration must be in whole blood rather than plasma. If plasma concentrations are measured, one must determine

Table 3-1

**Numerical Example of the Application of the Fick Principle
to the Calculation of Oxygen, Glucose, and Lactate Net Fluxes**

Experimental data
Uterine blood flow   = 1600 ml/min
Umbilical blood flow =   800 ml/min

	Maternal artery	Uterine vein	Umbilical vein	Umbilical artery
Oxygen				
(μmol/ml)	6.00	4.65	5.45	3.98
Glucose				
(μmol/ml)	2.80	2.62	1.20	1.08
Lactate				
(μmol/ml)	0.66	0.70	1.69	1.58

Calculations
Net fluxes to pregnant uterus from maternal blood (μmol/min)
Oxygen flux = 1600 × (6.00 − 4.65) = 2160
Glucose flux = 1600 × (2.80 − 2.62) =   288
Lactate flux = 1600 × (0.66 − 0.70) = −64

Net fluxes to fetal blood from placenta (μmol/min)
Oxygen flux = 800 × (5.45 − 3.98) = 1176
Glucose flux = 800 × (1.20 − 1.08) =   96
Lactate flux = 800 × (1.69 − 1.58) =   88

Uteroplacental and glucose consumption and lactate production (μmol/min)
Oxygen consumption = 2160 − 1176 = 984
Glucose consumption =   288 − 96   = 192
Lactate production   =   88 + 64   = 152

whether the substance under investigation is also carried by the red cells
and define the magnitude of the red cell–plasma exchange. If the substance of interest exists in blood in different chemical forms, large errors
can be introduced by an inappropriate choice of the method of analysis. A
classical case is oxygen, which is carried by blood in two forms—free and
bound to hemoglobin. Methods that measure only free oxygen (P_{O_2} measurements) cannot be used to measure blood oxygen content. In theory
estimates of blood oxygen content could be derived from P_{O_2} measurements if the oxyhemoglobin dissociation curve of each blood sample were
known. In practice, direct measurement of blood oxygen content or of the
oxygen carried by hemoglobin are much more reliable.

Blood has the capacity to metabolize certain molecules as it circulates
through an organ, thus altering the meaning of arteriovenous concentration differences. In most cases this is not a significant problem, but there
can be exceptions. An organ, for example, can be endowed with a lipase

that rapidly hydrolyzes blood lipids into fatty acids. The arteriovenous difference of fatty acids across this organ will represent the algebraic sum of fatty acids produced by the blood as well as those taken up by the organ. Under such conditions the organ could derive a significant amount of fatty acids from the blood without causing the venous concentration to be less than the arterial concentration.

The uterine and umbilical venous samples must represent the whole venous drainage of the uterine and umbilical circulations, respectively. In the case of the umbilical circulation this condition can be satisfied by placing the tip of the sampling catheter in the common umbilical vein. There is no common uterine venous drainage, however. In ewes carrying a single fetus, the tip of the uterine venous catheter can be placed in the large uterine vein of the pregnant horn, approximately 4 cm below the level of the ovary, on the assumption that the composition of the blood sampled at this site represents the composition of the whole uterine venous output. In single fetuses with placental cotyledons in both uterine horns, the validity of this assumption is supported by the observation that, in general, venous samples drawn simultaneously from the right and left uterine veins have virtually equal composition and yield comparable blood flow values. Exceptions are possible, however, in which case the metabolic exchange between pregnant uterus and maternal blood cannot be accurately quantified. In ewes carrying twins, the placental cotyledons of each twin tend to be confined to one uterine horn. Thus, by infusing the blood flow indicator in one fetus and by sampling the venous drainage of the uterine horn containing that fetus, it is possible to estimate blood flow and substrate fluxes to the uteroplacenta of one of the twins. In experiments with twins, the position of the placental cotyledons should be verified at autopsy.

Other methods of uterine blood flow determination (e.g., microsphere method and electromagnetic flow probes) have been used (see Chapter 8), but they are not as well suited for metabolic studies. The microsphere technique can provide accurate measurements of blood flow which are, however, limited to a few points in time. With this technique there is no assurance that the flow measurements do, in fact, represent the flow over the period in which the substrate concentrations were measured and that the preparation was in a steady state. A flow probe placed around one middle uterine artery is the instrument of choice for the continuous recording of flow. Therefore, flow probes have been used in preference to any other method for studies of the regulation of uterine blood flow. The uterus, however, is supplied with blood by several arteries so that measurements of blood flow through a single uterine artery do not provide adequate information about the total perfusion rate of the uteroplacenta.

Problems of accuracy in flow determinations and in blood sampling technique suggest caution in accepting estimates of metabolic rates that are made by using flow measurements in one group of animals and arteriovenous difference measurements in a second group of animals, especially if the two sets come from different laboratories.

Measurements of arteriovenous differences often represent the principal source of random error in the calculation of metabolic fluxes through an application of the Fick principle. There are two potential errors. One is introduced by the factors involved in obtaining the blood sample from a vessel. In chronically catheterized large animals the length of the catheter from the site of entry into the blood vessel to the outside of the mother can be quite long. If the catheter material is highly permeable to blood gases or the sample comes in contact with air, the oxygen and carbon dioxide content may change during sampling. Similarly, if the sample can only be withdrawn very slowly, there may be alterations in substrate concentrations in the blood after it leaves the vessel but before it is collected and preserved for analysis.

The second error relates to the "coefficient of extraction," that is, the percentage change in the concentration of a solute as the blood perfuses an organ. Table 3-2 lists representative coefficients of extraction across the umbilical circulation of the fetal lamb for some metabolic substrates. As one can see, it would be impossible to arrive at any precise estimate of urea excretion from the fetal circulation by an application of the Fick

Table 3-2

Coefficients of Extraction across Umbilical
Circulation of Fetal Lamb at 120 + Days
Gestation (Well-Nourished Ewes)

Substrate	Coefficient (%)
Oxygen	40
Glucose	10
Fructose	~1
Lactate	8
Pyruvate	undetectable
Urea	0.4
Free fatty acids	undetectable
Acetate	18
Glycerol	15
β-hydroxybutyrate	0–3
Acetoacetate	10–20
Neutral amino acids	3% for glycine up to 14 % for isoleucine
Basic amino acids	6% for histidine up to 21% for arginine

principle to the flux of urea since urea changes its concentration by only 0.4% as the blood perfuses the placenta. By contrast, the oxygen consumption of the fetus can be determined precisely since there is an approximate 40% change in oxygen content during placental perfusion. The amino acids represent a group of compounds of great interest in this regard since the coefficients of extraction for most amino acids are at the borderline of what can be measured with any reasonable precision. Figure 3-2 presents data from our laboratory for the arteriovenous differences of amino acids across the uterine circulation of the pregnant sheep (43). The coefficient of extraction for the neutral amino acids is approximately 6–8%, for the basic amino acids approximately 4–5%, and for the acidic amino acids unmeasurably small. For the purposes of this discussion it is instructive to compare phenylalanine and glycine. Both amino acids are extracted with an arteriovenous difference of approximately 4 μM. However, since the blood level of glycine is approximately ten times higher than that of phenylalanine, the coefficient of extraction of the two amino acids differ by tenfold, 0.6% for glycine and 6% for phenylalanine. Therefore, the high blood concentration makes detection of the glycine flux to the uterus (which, in absolute amounts, is about equal to that of phenylalanine) difficult to measure and has led some investigators to the unwar-

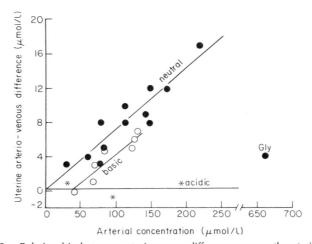

Figure 3-2: Relationship between arteriovenous differences across the uterine circulation and the arterial concentration of the amino acids. Linear regression lines are plotted, but the glycine value (mean arterial concentration 663 μM) was excluded from the regression analysis. ●, Neutral amino acids; ○, basic amino acids; ∗, acidic amino acids. From Holzman et al. (43).

ranted conclusion that there is no glycine uptake by the pregnant ovine uterus and that it must be synthesized entirely by the fetus and/or placenta.

It is clear, therefore, that the application of the Fick principle requires some attention to detail and to the peculiarities of the particular organ or tissue being studied in addition to attention to the lability of the substances whose concentrations are being determined. For the purpose of providing an example, we have outlined our approach to the measurement of the umbilical and uterine uptakes of oxygen, glucose and lactate. However, if one is studying other substances or studying the same compounds across other organs and tissues, it may necessitate changes in experimental design, although the same principles would apply in order to minimize errors in the estimation of substrate flux.

Relating Metabolic Fluxes to Tissue Weight

As illustrated by the numerical example in Table 3-1, measurements of metabolic fluxes can be reported in absolute terms, such as millimoles of oxygen or milligrams of glucose taken up each minute by the fetus via the umbilical circulation. To understand the physiologic meaning of such measurements, it is necessary to explore their relationship to each other and to other measurements. It is obvious, for example, that a statement such as "the fetus consumes 1 mmol/min of oxygen" would have little meaning if there was no information about the weight of the fetus. Hence, the common practice is to express the umbilical uptakes of oxygen and substrates as per kilogram of fetal body weight. This practice is based on the assumption that fetal metabolic rates are proportional to fetal mass. This is a fair assumption for fetuses of comparable age and physiologic conditions. However, it should be verified for each set of experimental data by regression analysis of metabolic rate versus fetal weight. Metabolic rates of the pregnant uterus have been reported either per kilogram of the combined weight of the fetus, placenta, and uterine wall (i.e., uterine weight minus the weight of fetal fluids) or per kilogram of fetus. This approach to the normalization of data can be useful, but it has limitations. In expressing the uptakes of oxygen and substrates by the pregnant uterus per unit weight of all its tissue components, one lumps together the placenta and fetus, which have different weight-specific metabolic rates. In expressing the net fluxes of metabolic substrates to the pregnant uterus per kilogram of fetus, one arbitrarily selects fetal weight to normalize metabolic rates, which in fact depend on the combined activity of fetus and placenta.

Metabolic Quotients

The relationship of fetal metabolic rate to fetal body weight is important when comparing fetuses of different species and when comparing fetal with postnatal life (see discussion of fetal oxygen consumption). Tissue mass, however, is not necessarily the best standard of reference in metabolic studies. Depending upon the nature of the problem, the use of tissue dry weight (10), DNA, or protein content may be preferable. For metabolic studies *in vivo,* the rate of oxygen consumption of the organism or organ under investigation is one of the most useful standards of reference. This is so for two main reasons. The first is that oxygen consumption defines the quantity of substrate that is needed to satisfy energy requirements. Therefore, if we compare the supply rate of a given substrate (e.g., glucose) with the oxygen consumption rate, we can judge whether the amount being supplied is large or small in relation to energy demands. The second reason is technical. If one measures the uptake of oxygen and other substrates by application of the Fick principle, neither measurement of blood flow nor of tissue mass is required for comparing substrate uptake rates with the oxygen consumption rate. For example, assume that both the glucose (R_G) and oxygen (R_{O_2}) uptakes by the fetus are measured. The two uptakes are related to umbilical venous–arterial concentration differences of glucose ($v_G - a_G$) and oxygen ($v_{O_2} - a_{O_2}$) and umbilical blood flow (f) by the equations

$$R_G = (v_G - a_G)f \tag{3-1}$$

and

$$R_{O_2} = (v_{O_2} - a_{O_2})f \tag{3-2}$$

It follows that the ratio of the two uptakes is equal to the ratio of the venous–arterial concentration differences:

$$R_G/R_{O_2} = (v_G - a_G)/(v_{O_2} - a_{O_2}) \tag{3-3}$$

Since substrate : oxygen uptake ratios can be measured without measuring blood flow, they can be defined more accurately and are easier to obtain than absolute or weight-specific uptakes. To facilitate the evaluation of substrate : oxygen uptake ratios, these ratios are generally reported as metabolic quotients. In the calculation of a metabolic quotient, the uptake of substrate is first converted to "oxygen equivalents," that is, the quantity of oxygen that is needed for complete oxidation to CO_2 and water, and then divided by the oxygen uptake. For example, in the calculation of glucose/oxygen quotients, the glucose concentration difference, expressed in millimoles per liter, is multiplied by six and then divided by the oxygen concentration difference, also expressed in millimoles per liter. Table 3-3 lists some of the common metabolites and the equations describing their complete oxidation. It is clear from this table that some of the difficulty in calculating net free fatty acid uptake by tissues, which may be consuming significant quantities of this substrate, stems from the fact that a relatively small uptake of free fatty acids can represent a very substantial contribution to the fuel requirements of the tissue, given the 20-fold difference in molar equivalents of oxygen and free fatty acids. If the metabolic quotient of a given substrate is consistently below 1.0, one can conclude that the uptake of that substrate cannot satisfy energy requirements and that other substrates must be used for that purpose. The metabolic quotients across a given circulation can be summed algebraically and compared with theoretical expectations (metabolic quotients can be either positive or negative since there can be either net uptake or net delivery of metabolites). For a nongrowing organ or organism, the theoretical expectation is that over a suitably long time period the sum of all metabolic quotients tends to 1.0. For a growing system, the sum of all metabolic quotients should be greater than 1.0, since there is both accretion and oxidation of substrates. How much greater than 1.0 this sum should be can be estimated from caloric accretion data.

A common misconception about metabolic quotients is that their validity depends upon the assumption that the substrate under consideration is completely oxidized to CO_2 and H_2O and that they are not as reliable as

Table 3-3

**Reference Table of Some Substrates and
Their Metabolic and Respiratory Quotients**

| | | Quotients | |
| | | Metabolic | |
Substrate	Equation	($\times$ substrate/oxygen)	Respiratory
Glucose	$C_6H_{12}O_6 + 6\ O_2 = 6\ CO_2 + 6\ H_2O$	6	1.0
Lactate	$C_3H_6O_3 + 3\ O_2 = 3\ CO_2 + 3\ H_2O$	3	1.0
Glycerol	$2\ C_3H_8O_3 + 7\ O_2 = 6\ CO_2 + 8\ H_2O$	3.5	0.86
Acetic acid	$C_2H_4O_2 + 2\ O_2 = 2\ CO_2 + 2\ H_2O$	2	1.0
Decanoic acid	$C_{10}H_{20}O_2 + 14\ O_2 = 10\ CO_2 + 10\ H_2O$	14	0.71
Palmitic acid	$C_{16}H_{32}O_2 + 23\ O_2 = 16\ CO_2 + 16\ H_2O$	23	0.70
Acetoacetate	$C_4H_6O_3 + 4\ O_2 = 4\ CO_2 + 3\ H_2O$	4	1.0
β-hydroxybutyrate	$2\ C_4H_8O_3 + 9\ O_2 = 8\ CO_2 + 8\ H_2O$	4.5	0.89

metabolic rates expressed per unit tissue mass. In reality, the main purpose of calculating metabolic quotients is to use the rate of oxidative metabolism as the standard of reference. The usefulness of this reference does not depend on detailed knowledge about the rate of oxidation of each substrate. Furthermore, the use of different reference standards gives the opportunity of evaluating metabolism from different viewpoints, each adding its own unique information.

Tracer Methodology

In recent years tracer methods have been applied extensively to studies of fetal metabolism. Unfortunately, several studies were based on conceptual and/or technical errors which preclude an effective use of the experimental data. It seems worthwhile, therefore, to discuss in some detail the application of tracer methodology to the study of fetal metabolism, using tracer glucose as an example.

Fetal Tracer Glucose Infusion. If tracer glucose (e.g., [^{14}C]glucose uniformly labeled) is infused at a constant rate into the fetal circulation until a steady state is attained, a concentration gradient for tracer glucose is established across the placenta from fetal to maternal blood, that is, in a direction opposite to the normal glucose gradient for tracee (i.e., unlabeled glucose). Figure 3-3 presents the average concentrations for tracer and tracee glucose in maternal and fetal arterial blood for a series of experiments in our laboratory in which [^{14}C]glucose was infused into the inferior vena cava of fetal lambs (36). Since the transplacental concentration gradients for tracer and tracee glucose are in opposite directions, there is a net flux of tracer glucose from fetus to mother while the net flux of tracee glucose continues from the maternal to the fetal compartment.

Thus, the tracer glucose infused into the fetus is partitioned into two net fluxes, one that enters fetal metabolism and another that exits the fetus prior to any participation in fetal metabolism. The latter flux can be measured by application of the Fick principle to the loss of tracer via the umbilical circulation. Once the tracer infusion rate is partitioned into its two components, we can use the component that represents net flux into fetal metabolism to estimate the rate of fetal glucose utilization. The standard assumption that is made in this estimate is that the tracer : tracee concentration ratio (specific activity) determines the tracer : tracee metabolic utilization ratio. Since the glucose-specific activity in the fetal tis-

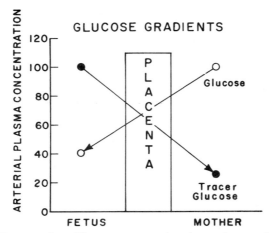

Figure 3-3: Concentration differences across the sheep placenta for tracer glucose [U-¹⁴C]glucose and unlabeled glucose after infusion of [¹⁴C]glucose into the fetal inferior vena cava. Note that the normal glucose gradient is from maternal to fetal circulation and that that determines a net glucose flux from mother to fetus. Since the tracer is infused into the fetus, its gradient is from fetal to maternal circulations and the net tracer flux is from fetus to mother.

sues that metabolize glucose is best represented by the fetal arterial specific activity, this activity is the one selected for calculating fetal glucose utilization. An example of calculations based on fetal tracer glucose infusion data is presented in Table 3-4A.

Table 3-4A

**Example of Calculation of Fetal Glucose
Utilization by Means of Tracer Glucose: Fetal Tracer Infusion**

Experimental data		
Umbilical blood flow	=	800 ml/min
Tracer glucose infusion rate	=	1,900,000 dpm/min

	Umbilical vein	Umbilical artery
Tracer glucose (dpm/ml)	9802	11,039
Tracee glucose (mg/ml)	0.213	0.194

Calculations		
Net tracer flux from fetus to placenta	$= 800(11,039 - 9802)$	= 989,600 dpm/ml
Net tracer flux into fetal metabolism	$= 1,900,000 - 989,600$	= 910,400 dpm/ml
Glucose specific activity in fetal pool	$= 11,039/0.194$	= 56,900 dpm/mg
Fetal glucose utilization rate	$= 910,400/56,900$	= 16.0 mg/min
Umbilical glucose uptake	$= 800(0.213 - 0.194)$	= 15.2 mg/min
Estimated fetal glucose production rate	$= 16.0 - 15.2$	= 0.8 mg/min

Under steady-state conditions, fetal glucose utilization should be either higher than or equal to the fetal uptake of glucose via the umbilical circulation, depending upon the presence or absence of glucose production within the fetus (fetal glucogenesis). Thus, by comparing in the same animal fetal glucose utilization with umbilical glucose uptake, one can estimate the magnitude of fetal glucose production (32). However, due to limitations in the accuracy of the different measurements that affect this estimate, the discrepancy between utilization and uptake would have to be fairly large and reproducible to be a reliable measure of fetal glucose production. Furthermore, such an experimental design does not distinguish glycogenolysis from gluconeogenesis (62).

Maternal Tracer Glucose Infusion. If tracer glucose is infused at a constant rate into the mother, we can visualize its disposal rate as partitioned into two net fluxes: (a) flux into the metabolism of the pregnant uterus and (b) flux into maternal metabolism (i.e., metabolism by maternal organs other than the pregnant uterus). The net tracer flux into the pregnant uterus can be measured by application of the Fick principle to the loss of tracer via the uterine circulation and subtracted from the maternal tracer infusion rate to calculate the flux of tracer into maternal metabolism. The two tracer metabolic fluxes can then be used in conjunction with measurements of maternal arterial specific activity to estimate separately the utilization rate of maternal glucose by the maternal organism and by the pregnant uterus. The partition of the utilization of a substrate between uterine and nonuterine tissues of the mother can be achieved in a relatively straightforward manner because the only complexity in the biologic preparation is the requirement of a sampling catheter in the main uterine venous drainage. The sampling of uterine venous blood under normal physiologic conditions has been accomplished successfully in the horse, cow, sheep, goat, guinea pig, and rabbit so that such studies are now feasible in those species.

If catheterization of the fetal side of the placental circulation is possible, as it is in sheep, then additional information can be derived by measuring the net entry rate of maternal glucose tracer into the fetus. Determination of the fetal tracer entry rate provides an estimate of fetal glucose utilization from the ratio of the entry rate divided by the glucose specific activity in fetal arterial blood. Table 3-4B gives an example of these calculations.

If the fetus and/or the placenta produce glucose, the specific activity of maternal tracer glucose in the fetal glucose pool should be less than that in the maternal glucose pool. Therefore, in an experiment in which tracer glucose is infused into the maternal circulation, equality of maternal and

Table 3-4B

**Example of Calculation of Fetal and Maternal Glucose
Utilization by Means of Tracer Glucose: Maternal Tracer Infusion**

Experimental data
  Uterine blood flow   =   1600 ml/min
  Umbilical blood flow   =   800 ml/min
  Tracer glucose infusion rate = 6,900,000 dpm/min

	Maternal artery	Uterine vein	Umbilical vein	Umbilical artery
Tracer glucose (dpm/ml)	23,708	22,285	10,228	9293
Tracee glucose (mg/ml)	0.500	0.470	0.219	0.200

Calculations
Net tracer flux into pregnant uterus	$1600(23{,}708 - 22{,}285)$	$= 2{,}277{,}000$ dpm/min
Net tracer flux into maternal metabolism	$6{,}900{,}000 - 2{,}277{,}000$	$= 4{,}623{,}000$ dpm/min
Net fetal tracer uptake	$800(10{,}228 - 9293)$	$= 748{,}000$ dpm/min
Glucose specific activity in maternal blood	$23{,}708/0.5$	$= 47{,}416$ dpm/mg
Glucose specific activity in fetal blood	$9293/0.2$	$= 46{,}465$ dpm/mg
Glucose utilization by mother	$4{,}623{,}000/47{,}416$	$= 97.5$ mg/min
Glucose utilization by fetus	$748{,}000/46{,}465$	$= 16.1$ mg/min
Glucose uptake by pregnant uterus	$1600(0.500 - 0.470)$	$= 48.0$ mg/min
Glucose uptake by fetus	$800(0.219 - 0.200)$	$= 15.2$ mg/min

fetal glucose-specific activities should imply that the glucose utilized by placenta and fetus is entirely of maternal origin. However, a discrepancy between maternal and fetal specific activities could be difficult to detect, even in the presence of a physiologically significant fetal glucose production rate. This condition prevails if the exchange of labeled and unlabeled glucose across the placenta is very rapid. For this reason, we must be cautious in interpreting maternal : fetal blood specific activity ratios. A ratio that is not significantly different from 1.0 does not exclude fetal production of the molecules under investigation. Conversely, a ratio that is significantly less than 1.0 unequivocally indicates fetal production but does not establish the magnitude of the production rate.

Potential Errors in Fetal Tracer Methodology

Analytic Techniques and Sampling Sites. Differences in the composition of maternal and fetal blood should be considered whenever an analytical method that was previously used in the study of postnatal life is used in fetal studies. For example, the blood of fetal sheep has a high fructose concentration. When the fetus receives labeled glucose there is a slow labeling of the fructose molecules. Consequently, the analytical techniques that are most frequently used in measuring the specific activity of glucose in adult blood are not suited for the analysis of fetal blood because these techniques do not discriminate between glucose and fructose.

In performing tracer experiments *in vivo,* the choice of infusion and sampling sites is often of critical importance. Katz (49) has directed attention to this problem for tracer experiments in postnatal life. Additionally, in designing fetal experiments one must take into consideration the effect of transplacental exchange upon specific activity measurements. For example, whenever tracer glucose is infused into the fetal inferior vena cava, umbilical venous specific activity is less than umbilical arterial specific activity because the tracer molecules carried by fetal blood to the placenta exchange rapidly with, and are diluted by, unlabeled glucose molecules entering the fetus from the mother.

Selection of Tracer Models. Tracer experiments *in vivo* provide the opportunity to calculate a rate that has been variously named "turnover," "replacement," "production," or "irreversible disposal" of the molecules under investigation. If the tracer is infused at a constant rate into the circulation and steady-state blood specific activity is attained, then the turnover rate is equal to the infusion rate : steady-state specific activity ratio. The turnover calculation serves to define a physicochemical property of the system, namely, how rapidly tracee molecules exit the infused pool to be replaced by molecules "new" to the pool. Since molecules can enter and exit a pool via completely different mechanisms—via random exchange with another pool (diffusional exchange), via excretion, and via metabolic processes—the physiologic meaning of turnover must be carefully investigated by a realistic modeling of the system. Failure to do so has resulted in substantial errors of interpretation (2). For example, we can refer to the data in Table 3-4A, which are representative of actual experimental data, and calculate the error involved in assuming that fetal glucose turnover represents the rate of fetal glucose metabolism. The turnover rate, calculated by dividing the fetal tracer infusion rate by the fetal arterial glucose-specific activity is 33.4 mg/min, whereas the fetal glucose metabolic rate is 16.0 mg/min. Thus, by assuming that turnover equals metabolic rate, an investigator would overestimate fetal glucose metabolic rate by approximately a factor of two. This large discrepancy is due to the fact that fetal glucose turnover includes both fetal metabolic rate and the exchange of glucose molecules at the placental–fetal blood interface.

To investigators with a good understanding of tracer methodology, the misinterpretation of fetal turnover rate, although fairly common, may seem a trivial and easily avoidable mistake. However, errors of interpretation are possible even when the system is analyzed by means of fairly sophisticated models. After realizing that some of the tracer glucose infused into the fetus enters maternal blood to be metabolized by maternal tissues, some investigators modeled maternal and fetal blood as two separate glucose pools that exchange glucose reversibly (two-pool reversible model) (42). This model predicts that by infusing two different types of tracer glucose separately into the mother and into the fetus, and by measuring the steady-state specific activities of both tracers in maternal and fetal blood, one can calculate both maternal and fetal glucose utilization rates. When we tested this model experimentally, however, we found that it overestimates by approximately 60% the rate of fetal glucose metabolism and that it overestimates by approximately 16% the net rate of glucose exit from the maternal glucose pool through routes other than the pregnant uterus (36). The error of interpretation, in this case, is the assumption implicit in the two-pool model that maternal and fetal blood are separated by a membrane that does not metabolize glucose. Given this assumption, the model partitions the glucose utilized by the whole system (i.e., mother, uteroplacenta, and fetus) so that a fraction of uteroplacental glucose utilization is assigned to the fetus and a fraction assigned to the mother. Figure 3-4 contrasts actual maternal, uteroplacental, and fetal

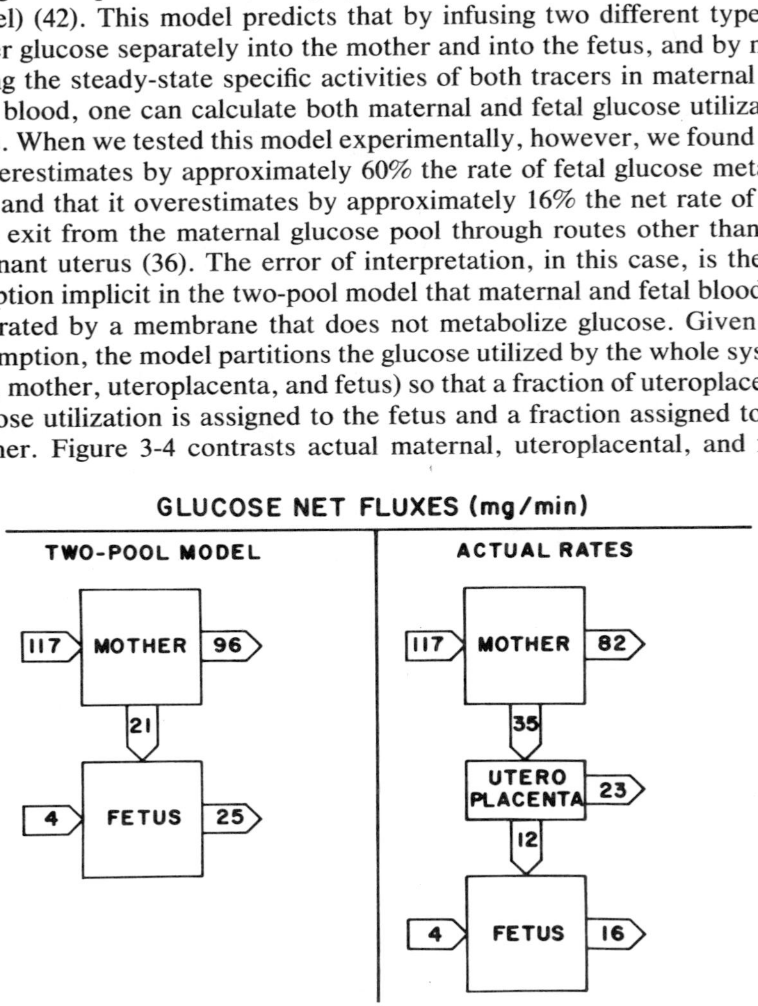

GLUCOSE NET FLUXES (mg/min)

Figure 3-4: Calculations of maternal and fetal glucose utilization rates by means of tracer methodology can be in error if the tracer model used in the calculations does not represent the actual system. A two-pool model of maternal–fetal glucose exchange overestimates fetal utilization by a large margin because it attributes to the fetus a large fraction of the uteroplacental glucose utilization. Data taken from Ref. 36.

glucose utilization rates with how the two-pool model views the utilization of glucose in the system.

UTERINE AND UMBILICAL OXYGEN UPTAKES

Several investigators have measured oxygen uptakes by the pregnant uterus and by the umbilical circulation of sheep separately using various techniques. These uptakes have also been measured simultaneously by the method illustrated in Figure 3-1. An example of the results of simultaneous measurements is given in Table 3-5. Note that the fetal uptake of oxygen via the umbilical circulation is considerably less than the uterine uptake, in other words, the tissues interposed between the uterine and umbilical circulations consume oxygen at a rapid rate.

There is general agreement that in the last month of pregnancy the normal oxygen uptake of fetal lambs is 6–8 ml_{STP}/kg/min body weight (or 0.26 to 0.36 mmol/kg/min). This information is of basic physiologic interest because the normal rate of fetal oxygen consumption is a measure of the rate of fetal energy metabolism. Although the caloric equivalents represented by 1 liter of oxygen consumption will vary depending upon the mix of carbohydrates, fats, and proteins used as fuel, the range is small (from 4.7 to 5.0 $kcal/liter_{STP}$ O_2). Furthermore, it is known that the fetal lamb consumes a diet of carbohydrates and amino acids, so that a 4.9 $kcal/liter_{STP}$ O_2 figure can be used to convert fetal oxygen consumption into calories without introducing any appreciable error. Therefore, we can estimate that the level of fetal energy metabolism in sheep is approximately 42–56 kcal/kg/day.

Fetal oxygen consumption rates have been measured in species other than sheep, and these results are summarized in Table 3-6. These results should be considered with caution because the techniques that were used

Table 3-5

**Simultaneously Measured Uterine and
Umbilical Oxygen Uptakes in Nine Ewes[a]**

	Fetal weight (kg)	Uterine O_2 uptake (mmol/min)	Umbilical O_2 uptake (mmol/min)	Uteroplacental O_2 utilization (mmol/min)
	4.03	2.16	1.18	0.98
(±SEM)	(±0.29)	(±0.15)	(±0.06)	(±0.13)

[a] From Meschia *et al.* (57).

and the state of the preparation may have introduced errors that cannot be easily detected in any single set of experiments. Nevertheless, in most species there has been some validation of these estimates. For example, the fetal guinea pig data, which were published by Bohr (17) in 1900, agree with a more recent study by Moll *et al.* (58), according to which the guinea pig uterus consumes oxygen at the rate of 8.8 ml/kg/min. Moll *et al.* employed an interesting approach that is similar in principle to the approach originally used by Bohr. They developed a technique that enabled the uterine circulation of unanesthetized pregnant guinea pigs to be occluded briefly from the outside, while the maternal oxygen consumption rate was measured continuously. The oxygen consumption of the gravid uterus was estimated from the decrease in maternal oxygen consumption during the occlusion.

The most interesting aspect of the comparative data in Table 3-6 is the indication that the rates of fetal oxygen consumption per unit of weight are quite similar in fetuses of different species despite very large differences in body size. There is a 300-fold difference in body mass between the guinea pig fetus and bovine fetus at term. This similarity is in sharp contrast with the well-established fact that in adult mammals the resting oxygen consumption rate is not proportional to body weight but to the body weight raised to a fractional exponent, which is approximately equal to 0.75 (51). Physiologic parameters that are linked to the rate of energy metabolism, such as cardiac output and heart rate, also show a strong influence of body size. Heart rate is much higher in small than in large adult mammals; for example, rates are as high as 1300 beats/min in the small shrew and as low as 15 beats/min in whales. As discussed more fully in Chapter 7 (on fetal circulation), the comparative study of fetal heart rate shows that this parameter is much less dependent on body size among fetuses than among adults, thus lending support to the notion that

Table 3-6

**Weight-Specific Oxygen Consumption Rates
of Fetuses in Species of Different Sizes**

	O_2 Consumption (ml_{STP}/kg/min)	Reference
Horse	7.0	69
Cattle	6.7	21
Sheep	7.0	6
Man	8.0	65
Rhesus monkey	7.0	9
Guinea pig	8.8	17, 58

weight-specific oxygen consumption rate is much less variable in prenatal than in postnatal life.

The hypothesis that fetal metabolic rate expressed on a weight-specific basis may be fairly similar among mammals despite large differences in fetal birthweight has important implications in the comparative physiology of reproduction. As already discussed in Chapter 1, allometric relationships have been described between birthweight and maternal weight in mammals, showing an inverse relationship between maternal size and the fetal : maternal weight ratio (Chapter 1, Figure 1-3).

For mammals in general, Leitch *et al.* (52) derived the equation $F = 0.54M^{0.83}$ and Leutenegger (54) found $F = 0.12M^{0.7}$ for simian primates, where F and M are the total fetal weight at term and the prepregnancy maternal weight in kilograms, respectively. Both equations imply that smaller mammals produce a larger total fetal mass per kilogram of maternal body than larger mammals. If we compare fetal : maternal ratios for both weights and oxygen consumption, we can see the advantage to the smaller mammals of a weight-specific fetal metabolic rate that is low in comparison to the maternal weight-specific metabolic rate. Table 3-7 presents estimates in the three species in which sufficient data are available for calculation—the guinea pig, sheep, and cow. The fetal size ranges from approximately 80 g in the guinea pig fetus at term to 25 kg in the calf. The litter size is assumed to be one for the cow and sheep and four for the guinea pig. Although the fetal : maternal weight ratios differ from 6.25% in the cow to 32% in the guinea pig (a fivefold difference), the fetal : maternal oxygen consumption ratios are similar: 15% in the cow versus 23% in the guinea pig (only a 50% higher ratio in the guinea pig). Clearly, one of the physiologic reasons the guinea pig can carry a large fetal mass to term is

Table 3-7

Comparison of Fetal : Maternal Ratios for Weight
and O_2 Consumption Rate in Three Species

		Fetal mass (F)	Maternal mass (M)	Fetal : maternal weight ratio (%)	Fetal : maternal O_2 consumption ratio[a] (%)
Jersey cow	(kg)	25 /	400 =	6.25	6.25 × 6.72 / 2.7 = 15.6
Western sheep	(kg)	4.5 /	50 =	9.00	9.00 × 7.00 / 3.8 = 16.6
Guinea pig	(g)	4 × 80 /	1000 =	32.00	32.00 × 8.80 / 12.2 = 23.1

[a] The fetal : maternal oxygen consumption ratio ($\dot{V}_{O_2}$ of fetus ÷ $\dot{V}_{O_2}$ of mother) is obtained by multiplying the fetal : maternal weight ratio times the weight-specific oxygen consumption ratio of the maternal and fetal organism.

that, on a weight-specific basis, the oxygen demands of the fetus are relatively small in comparison to the oxygen demands of the maternal organism.

Comparative data for fetal oxygen consumption rates shed light on two issues around which there has been considerable debate. The first is whether the intensity of fetal energy metabolism is high or low in relation to maternal energy metabolism. The answer seems to be that the fetus is a relatively "cold spot" metabolically if the mother is a small mammal and a relatively "hot spot" if the mother is a large mammal. This interspecies difference is not due to any fundamental difference among fetuses, but rather to the marked influence of body size on the energy metabolism of the maternal organism (4, 6). The second issue is whether the transition from intra- to extrauterine life at birth requires an increase in oxygen consumption. Again, there is no single answer that is valid for all species. The mature fetal lamb has an oxygen consumption rate about equal to that of a resting adult mammal of the same size. Therefore, no large change in basal oxygen consumption is required at birth for a successful adaptation to a thermoneutral environment. It is even possible that in very large mammals there is a small decrease of oxygen consumption after birth. Comline and Silver (21) have reported an oxygen consumption in an un-anesthetized, unstressed fetal calf of 6.72 ± 0.23 ml/kg/min, whereas Thompson and Bell (82) reported oxygen consumptions in two 12-hr-old calves of 5.8 and 5.0 ml/kg/min, respectively. By contrast, in the smallest mammals the fetus probably has a much lower metabolic rate than that required for independent life. Hence, postnatal adaptation would require a major increase in metabolic rate. Measurements of fetal and neonatal heart rate in different species support the concept that body size has a profound influence on the metabolic changes of birth (56).

FETAL METABOLIC BALANCE

The fetus uses the uptake of nutrients via the umbilical circulation to fulfill two major requirements: (a) accretion, to build new tissues and to increase its storage of substrates (68), and (b) oxidation, to fuel energy metabolism. The rate at which the fetus builds new tissues and increases substrate storage can be estimated from data on fetal growth and body composition. The rate of energy metabolism can be estimated from fetal oxygen consumption. If both rates are expressed in kilocalories per day, they can be compared directly and summed to calculate the total flux of calories from placenta to fetus. The fetal caloric and carbon balances are presented schematically in Figure 3-5. Sufficient data are available to

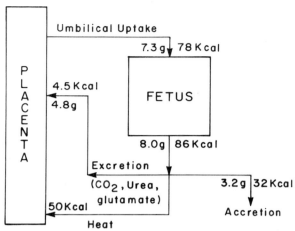

Figure 3-5: A diagram of the energy and carbon balance for the fetal lamb in the last 20% of gestation. The data for this calculation were derived from studies in the authors' laboratories from two general groups of studies: (a) studies of the net umbilical uptake and excretion of compounds and (b) studies of the body composition of the fetus at various gestational ages. Discrepancies between input and output reflect experimental error and/or incomplete information about the placental exchange of nutrients and excreta. The numerical data are from Table 3-8.

estimate the caloric balance of a sheep fetus in late gestation (Table 3-8). For example, at 130 days gestation the fetal lamb accumulates approximately 32 kcal/kg/day in the form of new tissue and uses approximately 50 kcal/kg/day to sustain its oxidative metabolism and excretes approximately 4.5 kcal/kg/day in the form of urea and glutamate. Hence, its nutritional requirements are approximately 86.5 kcal/kg/day. This calculation demonstrates the quantitative importance of oxidative metabolism in the ovine fetus. In other species the relative importance of anabolic and catabolic processes in determining total fetal metabolic requirements may be substantially different because there are marked interspecies differences in fetal growth rate.

The concept of metabolic balance is an important tool that can be applied to the analysis of every aspect of fetal metabolism despite its dynamic and complex nature. Often, it is by quantitatively matching the inputs and outputs of substrates that one can determine the self consistency and margin of error of the available information. To construct a metabolic balance may require the use of fetal growth curves and body composition, as in the case of caloric balance, or it may require tracer methodology. Furthermore, the balance study may be focused on long-

Table 3-8

Experimental Data on the Carbon and Energy Balance of a 130-Day-Old Sheep Fetus

	Carbon balance (g/kg/day)	Energy balance (kcal/kg/day)
Accumulating in carcass	3.15	32.0
Excretion		
As CO_2	4.38	0
As urea	0.16	2.0
As glutamate	0.30	2.5
Heat production	0	50.0
Total requirement	7.99	86.5
Umbilical uptake		
As glucose	1.8	16.6
As lactate	1.4	14.0
As acetate	0.2	2.5
As amino acids	3.9	44.8
Total entry	7.3	77.9

term or short-term processes. The following brief discussion of fetal carbon and fetal glucose carbon balance illustrates these differences.

In considering the fetal carbon balance (Figure 3-5), the main issues we are concerned with are (a) quantifying the diet of the fetus, that is, the umbilical uptake of all forms of carbon; (b) the irreversible loss of carbon from the fetal compartment, principally in the form of CO_2 excretion from the umbilical circulation into the placenta; and (c) the rate of carbon accretion in the body determined from a growth curve and serial whole body analyses during fetal life. The first two of these rates can be defined fairly accurately for a population of fetuses and for relatively long periods (days or weeks). This output information can then be compared with umbilical substrate uptakes to verify whether the sum of the substrate uptakes matches reasonably well the output data. A calculation of carbon and energy balance for the fetal lamb in the last month of gestation is presented in Table 3-8.

By contrast, when we attempt to evaluate the fetal glucose carbon balance (Figure 3-6), tracer methodology is required to measure fetal glucose utilization and the conversion of glucose carbon to CO_2 carbon. Tracer methodology gives a relatively short-term window into metabolic pathways; that is, if the study is carried out over several hours, we obtain input and output data and a description of the partition of glucose carbon between accretion (e.g., into fat and glycogen) and CO_2 production for

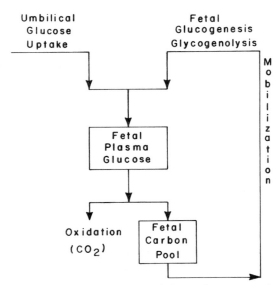

Figure 3-6: A diagram of fetal glucose carbon balance; the entries and exits from the fetal plasma glucose pool are shown. Fetal glucose production can be estimated from the difference between simultaneous measurements of umbilical glucose uptake and fetal glucose utilization.

that period alone. Over a longer period (e.g., several days) the carbon from glucose which has been incorporated into various carbon stores might well be remobilized and contribute significantly to subsequent CO_2 production. However, an important advantage of glucose carbon balance studies is that they can be carried out in individual fetuses comparing both umbilical uptake and fetal utilization and do not require any assumption about the rate of fetal growth at the time of the study.

GLUCOSE METABOLISM

A measurement of the umbilical uptake of oxygen is also a measurement of the rate of fetal oxygen utilization since there are no appreciable stores of oxygen within the fetus. This interpretation does not apply to the umbilical uptake of glucose nor is this necessarily true for any other substance having the potential to be synthesized and/or stored within the fetus. One cannot assume that a measurement of umbilical glucose uptake is equal to the rate of fetal glucose utilization. However, the umbilical glucose uptake does represent the exogenous supply or dietary supply of glucose to the fetus and as such is an important measurement in the study of fetal metabolism. Figure 3-6 presents a diagram of fetal glucose exit and entry into the glucose pool of the fetus. At present, fetal glucose uptake and utilization have been investigated extensively in only one species, the sheep. Therefore, we shall use the information about glucose metabolism in the ovine fetus as the standard of comparison to which data in other species are related for interpretation.

Uterine and Umbilical Glucose Uptakes

Under normal physiologic conditions the glucose uptake by the pregnant uterus of near term ewes carrying a single fetus is approximately 50 mg/min and approximately three times as high as the net flux of glucose from placenta to fetus (Table 3-9). Several comparisons of umbilical glucose and oxygen uptakes have shown that the umbilical glucose/oxygen quotient is significantly less than 1.0. In a study of well-nourished ewes it was 0.65 (95% confidence limits 0.54–0.74) (6). These data establish three important aspects of fetal glucose metabolism in sheep: (a) the placenta metabolizes a very large fraction of the glucose that the mother delivers to the pregnant uterus, (b) glucose is a quantitatively important fetal nutrient, and (c) the amount of glucose supplied to the fetus by the placenta is substantially less than the amount of substrate needed to sustain fetal energy metabolism even under optimal physiologic conditions. As discussed later, the oxidative metabolism of fetal lambs is fueled by several metabolites in addition to glucose, primarily amino acids and lactate.

Umbilical glucose/oxygen quotients have been measured in several species, as shown in Table 3-10. In all species studied thus far the quotient has been less than 1.0, implying that substrates other than glucose must be used as fuel by the fetus in all these species as well. The highest quotient reported thus far (0.8) is that estimated across the umbilical circulation of the human fetus. However, since such data were collected under the

Table 3-9

Simultaneously Measured Uterine and Umbilical Glucose Uptakes in 12 Ewes[a]

	Fetal weight (kg)	Uterine glucose uptake (mmol/min)	Umbilical glucose uptake (mmol/min)	Uteroplacental glucose utilization (mmol/min)
	4.53	0.288	0.082	0.206
(±SEM)	(±0.38)	(±0.020)	(±0.008)	(±0.016)

[a] From Meschia et al. (57).

Table 3-10

Umbilical Glucose/
Oxygen Quotients

Species	Quotient	Reference
Humans	0.80	60
Sheep	0.45	83
Cows	0.57	69
Horses	0.69	69

stress of labor and delivery, whereas those in other species were collected under chronic steady-state conditions before parturition had begun, the values are not comparable. Presumably for the same reasons, the variance of the glucose/oxygen quotients in humans was quite large. Despite these reservations, it would not be surprising to find a higher umbilical glucose/oxygen quotient in humans than in ruminants such as sheep and cows for several reasons. The first reason has to do with body composition of the fetus. The human newborn, in contrast to most other primates

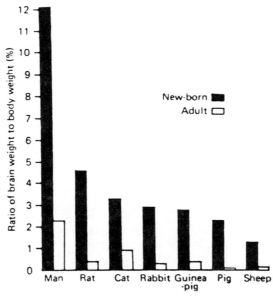

Figure 3-7: Ratio of brain:body weight in selected newborn and adult mammals. From Cross (22).

and to the lamb and calf, has a high concentration of body fat at birth with most of this fat represented by white fat depots. Since fat is approximately 78% carbon, this difference in fetal body composition dictates a much higher carbon accretion rate for the same rate of increase in fetal weight (75). Some of this carbon for lipogenesis may come to the fetus in the form of glucose. The human placenta is permeable to free fatty acids, but their estimated rates of placental transport appear to be inadequate to account for the total fat depots of the infant. A second reason for increased glucose requirement in the human fetus compared to the sheep stems from the differences in brain : body weight ratios in the two species. Since the brain of the fetus is a major site of glucose consumption (see Chapter 5), the much higher brain : body weight ratio in humans (Figure 3-7) increases the fetal glucose requirement in this species.

A third reason why the umbilical glucose/oxygen quotient may indeed be higher in humans stems from differences in placental permeability to glucose. Figure 3-8 compares published data for fetal and maternal arterial glucose concentrations in several species. It is clear that in all species studied the fetal glucose concentration is lower than that in the maternal

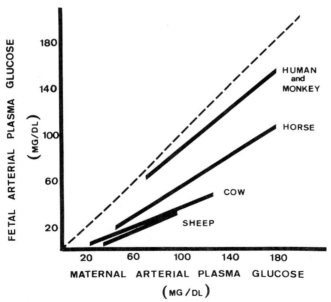

Figure 3-8: The relationship of fetal arterial plasma glucose concentration to maternal arterial plasma glucose concentration for humans (20a), monkey (20b), horse (69), cow (69), and sheep (70, 74). Reproduced from Ref. 5.

circulation. However, in humans and other primates the transplacental difference in glucose concentration is much smaller than in sheep and cows, suggesting a higher placental permeability to glucose in the hemochorial placenta. It should be noted that the slope of the regression line relating fetal to maternal arterial glucose concentrations is not parallel to that of an identity line in any of the species presented in Figure 3-8, but instead is significantly less. As maternal glucose concentration increases, the concentration difference across the placenta increases. In sheep and presumably in other species, this type of relationship is due to umbilical glucose uptake varying in direct relation to maternal glucose concentration. To our knowledge, the only report describing a higher glucose concentration in the fetus compared to that in the mother is by Woods *et al.* (89) for guinea pigs. However, these data were collected under acute, non-steady-state conditions, and it is likely that the results simply reflect increased glycogenolysis in the fetus secondary to catecholamine release rather than being an accurate reflection of normal transplacental gradients.

One of the most interesting results of studies of umbilical glucose uptake in chronic sheep preparations has been the demonstration that the net flux of glucose from placenta to fetus varies markedly as a function of maternal nutrition. In pregnant ewes deprived of food, umbilical glucose uptake decreases rapidly to approximately half its normal value by the second day of fasting, despite insignificant changes in fetal oxygen uptake. As a consequence, the umbilical glucose/oxygen quotient in fasting pregnant ewes can be quite small (mean = 0.3). The decrease of umbilical glucose uptake with fasting is triggered by maternal hypoglycemia and involves the interplay of placental glucose transfer mechanisms and fetal mechanisms of glucose regulation.

Placental Glucose Transfer Mechanisms

The observation that the normal flux of glucose from placenta to fetus is associated with a concentration difference between maternal and fetal plasma suggests the hypothesis that placental glucose transfer is by diffusion and that the glucose concentration must be lower in the fetus than in the mother in order to drive glucose across the placenta from the uterine to the umbilical circulation. This suggestion has been verified by experiments of fetal glucose infusion. If the normal glucose concentration difference across the placenta is decreased toward zero by elevating the fetal concentration of glucose, the net placenta to fetus glucose flux decreases and becomes negative. However, the transplacental diffusion of glucose is a more complex process than the passive diffusion of inert molecules for two main reasons: (a) the placental transfer of glucose is carrier mediated, and (b) the placental barrier has a high rate of glucose utilization.

Stacey et al. (79) demonstrated that in sheep the placental clearance of 3-O-methyl-D-glycopyranose (3-MDG), a metabolically inert analog of glucose, is much greater than that of molecules of similar size and solubility characteristics. Furthermore, they demonstrated that the transplacental diffusion rate of 3-MDG is inhibited by fetal hyperglycemia. Both findings indicate that the transplacental diffusion of glucose is mediated by saturable carriers that bind glucose molecules selectively. Experiments with isolated guinea pig placenta (66) have led to the same conclusion.

The hypothesis of carrier-mediated transfer was first proposed by Widdas in 1952 (88). Widdas suggested that the rate of diffusion of glucose from placenta to fetus (R_G) is determined by the intraplacental concentration gradient of a glucose–carrier complex, which is in reversible equilibrium with maternal and fetal plasma glucose at the maternal and fetal surfaces of the placenta. From this hypothesis, Widdas deduced the following equation of placental glucose transfer, which we have written in the familiar notation of Michaelis–Menton kinetics:

$$R_G = \dot{V}_{max} \left(\frac{A_G}{A_G + K_m} - \frac{a_G}{a_G + K_m} \right) \tag{3-4}$$

where $\dot{V}_{max}$ expresses the maximal flux of glucose, K_m is the concentration of glucose at which the carriers are half saturated, and A_G and a_G are the glucose concentrations in maternal and fetal arterial plasma, respectively. A major assumption, which is implicit in the Widdas equation, is that the placenta does not metabolize glucose. In reality, as we have seen, the placenta consumes glucose at a rapid rate. Furthermore, fetal blood is the source of a large fraction of the glucose molecules that are consumed by the placenta. Experiments in which two types of labeled glucose were infused simultaneously into mother and fetus have shown that the fetal glucose pool contributes approximately 40% of the glucose that is metabolized by the placenta (36).

To account for the hindrance that placental metabolism imposes upon the transfer of glucose from mother to fetus, it is necessary to add a negative term to the right side of the Widdas equation:

$$R_G = \dot{V}_{max} \left(\frac{A_G}{A_G + K_m} - \frac{a_G}{a_G + K_m} \right) - r_G \tag{3-5}$$

where r_G represents the net transfer of glucose from fetus to placenta that would occur if maternal and fetal plasma had equal glucose concentrations.

Experiments (74) in eight fetal sheep with mean body weight of 4.95 kg and placental weight of 0.317 kg estimated the placental K_m for glucose to be 70 mg/dl and provided the following empirical relationship between placenta to fetus glucose transfer and the arterial concentrations of glucose:

$$R_G = 209 \left(\frac{A_G}{A_G + 70} - \frac{a_G}{a_G + 70} \right) - 35.3 \qquad (3\text{-}6)$$

where R_G is in milligrams per minute and A_G and a_G are the arterial concentrations of glucose in maternal (A) and fetal (a) plasma, expressed as milligrams per deciliter. The y intercept is a negative term (-35.3 mg/min) comparable in magnitude to normal umbilical glucose uptake and therefore physiologically significant. For example, a fetus requiring 20 mg/min of glucose at a maternal arterial plasma glucose concentration of 70 mg/dl, will have a plasma arterial glucose concentration of 22 mg/dl. Hypothetically, in the absence of placental glucose consumption (y intercept = 0), the same fetus would have a glucose concentration of 47 mg/dl. This analysis leads to the conclusion that placental metabolism contributes significantly to the physiologic hypoglycemia of the fetal lamb, with fetal and placental metabolism competing for glucose.

The Widdas equation and its more recent modification are based on the hypothesis that the transfer rate of glucose from placenta to fetus depends primarily on the concentration of glucose in maternal and fetal arterial plasma and on the properties of the placental membrane (e.g., number of glucose carriers and metabolic activity) rather than on the rate of placental perfusion by maternal and fetal blood. This hypothesis has been tested recently on models of placental transfer (74) and by experimental observations on the effect of restricting uterine blood flow on fetal glucose (unpublished observations). Both approaches have validated the hypothesis by demonstrating that variations of maternal placental perfusion have a negligible effect on both fetal glucose uptake and concentration as long as the mother is normoglycemic and the variations in perfusion do not cause severe fetal hypoxia.

An important question is the extent to which placental glucose transfer mechanisms are under hormonal regulation. No studies have been performed addressing the question of chronic regulation. Acute regulation of placental transport by insulin has been tested through experiments in which insulin was infused into either the mother or the fetus while the concentration of blood glucose in the infused organism was kept at control levels by a variable infusion rate of glucose (glucose clamp technique) (37, 39). Under these experimental conditions, both the uterine and umbilical uptake of glucose did not increase significantly, indicating that placental glucose utilization and transfer are insensitive to short-term variations in the level of maternal and fetal insulin. In view of this result, the function of the insulin receptors that have been described in the placentas of several species needs further investigation.

Fetal Glucose Utilization and Production

At steady state in which both fetal glucose concentration and volume of distribution are constant, fetal glucose utilization will be equal to glucose entry from two sources: the exogenous supply of glucose to the fetus determined by the umbilical glucose uptake, and the endogenous production of glucose:

$$\text{Fetal glucose utilization} = \text{exogenous glucose uptake}$$
$$+ \text{endogenous glucose production}$$

In well-nourished ewes, fetal glucose utilization and the uptake of exogenous glucose are virtually equal, indicating that fetal glucogenesis is not an important source of fetal glucose (32). A low rate of glucogenesis in the fetal lamb with the mother in the fed state is supported by our studies of lactate turnover in the fetus (77) in which a slow rate of glucose labeling was observed when [^{14}C]lactate was infused at a constant rate into the fetus (fetal glucose-specific activity was approximately 3.3% of the fetal lactate-specific activity). During fasting, maternal hypoglycemia is accompanied by both a decrease in the fetal uptake of glucose via the umbilical circulation and a decrease in the fetal glucose utilization rate (Figure 3-9) (38). However, fetal glucose utilization does not decrease as

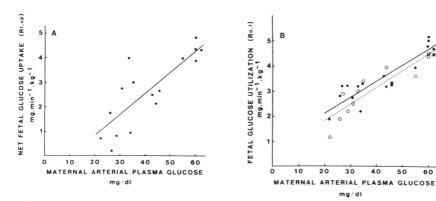

Figure 3-9:   A. Fetal glucose uptake versus maternal arterial plasma glucose concentration ($y = 0.09x - 0.96$, $r = 0.82$, $p < 0.001$) (40). B. Fetal glucose utilization versus maternal arterial plasma glucose. [U-^{14}C]glucose tracer values from a fetal infusion (●, ——) ($y = 0.062x + 0.91$, $r = 0.90$, $p < 0.001$) and [6-^{3}H]glucose tracer values from an infusion of tracer into mother (○, ————) ($y = 0.067x + 0.46$, $r = 0.89$, $p < 0.001$) (38).

much as the uptake of exogenous glucose, implying that at low levels of umbilical glucose uptake the fetus increases its endogenous production of glucose. Figure 3-10 presents fetal glucose utilization and production rates as a function of umbilical glucose uptake. These observations emphasize the importance of comparing rates of net substrate flux into the umbilical circulation with rates of utilization in the same animal preparation if an internal consistency to metabolic data is to be obtained. Some of the confusion in the literature regarding the question of whether there is

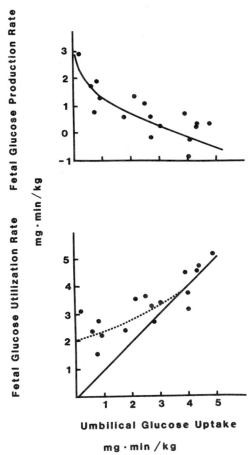

Figure 3-10: The relationship between umbilical glucose uptake (the exogenous supply of glucose to the fetus) and fetal glucose utilization and production rates. As the supply of glucose to the fetus from the placenta decreases, fetal glucose utilization rate does not decrease proportionately but is sustained by an increasing fetal glucose production rate. Data from Ref. 38.

an appreciable rate of fetal glucogenesis may simply reflect differences in the nutritional state of the animals at the time of study as well as some of the errors in either technique or experimental design discussed earlier (63).

In summary, the fetal lamb exhibits a low rate of glucogenesis relative to its rate of glucose utilization in the fed state and a higher rate during maternal fasting or starvation. These general characteristics seem to be true for at least one other species—the rat. Girard *et al.* (30) described equal specific activities of glucose in the fetal and maternal circulations of the rat when labeled glucose is infused into the maternal circulation with the rat in the fed state, implying little or no glucogenesis under these conditions. Goodner and Thompson (31) reported a ratio of 0.76 in the fed state. By contrast, when the pregnant rat was starved for four days, the ratio of fetal to maternal specific activity decreased from 1.0 in the fed state to 0.64 in the fasted state in Girard's study and from 0.76 to 0.58 in Goodner's studies (Table 3-11). Considering the duration of the fasts, this is unlikely to be due to glycogenolysis.

The chain of events relating fetal glucose utilization and production to maternal glucose concentration involves the regulation of fetal metabolism by fetal insulin. Variations of maternal glucose cause variations in the transfer rate of glucose across the placenta and in the level of fetal plasma glucose. Changes in fetal glucose concentration alter the secretory rate of fetal insulin, which in turn controls fetal glucose utilization and production.

The existence of a regulatory loop interrelating fetal glucose and fetal insulin has been demonstrated by several experiments. In pregnant ewes subjected to a cycle of feeding, fasting, and refeeding, there was a positive correlation of plasma insulin and glucose in both mother and fetus (Figure 3-11). Since the ovine placenta is virtually impermeable to insulin, the insulin measured in fetal plasma is of fetal origin. The slopes of the regression lines relating insulin to glucose were similar in mother and fetus, but the intercepts were different, indicating that in fetal life the glucose regu-

Table 3-11

Fetal : Maternal Blood-Specific
Activity Ratios during Maternal
Tracer Glucose Infusion

Species	Fed	Fasted	Reference
Rat	0.76	0.58	31
Rat	1.0	0.64	30
Sheep	0.98	0.92	38

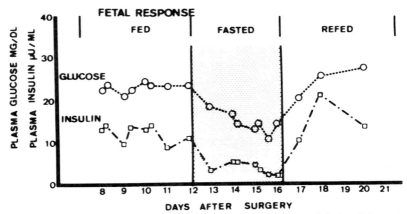

Figure 3-11: Fetal glucose and insulin responses to maternal fasting (61).

latory mechanism is set to control plasma glucose at a lower level than in postnatal life. Direct evidence for a control of fetal glucose concentration upon fetal insulin secretion was provided by experiments demonstrating that the infusion of glucose into the fetus elicits an insulin response (Figure 3-12) (3, 14, 61). Finally, experiments in which insulin was infused into fetal lambs demonstrated that fetal hyperinsulinemia increases the rate of utilization of glucose by fetal tissues (19, 39, 73).

Maternal Glucose Metabolism

Maternal glucose turnover rates have been measured in several species, coupled with measurements of maternal glucose concentration changes during pregnancy. It appears that a general characteristic of the pregnant state in mammals is a gradual decrease in maternal arterial glucose concentrations. Figure 3-13 presents data on maternal arterial glucose concentration versus gestational age for humans, rabbits, and guinea pigs. While the rate of decline is different among the species, there is a consistent pattern implying a new set point for maternal glucose concentration during pregnancy. This should not be interpreted as simply reflecting increasing caloric requirements of the conceptus in late gestation since the mother could easily increase food intake to accommodate those demands.

The glucose turnover rate during pregnancy tends to increase as maternal weight increases with growth of the conceptus, but the weight-specific turnover rate may not change significantly in some species. Table 3-12 compares the weight-specific turnover rates during pregnancy in several

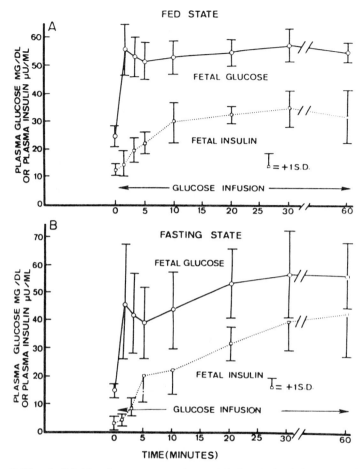

Figure 3-12: A. Fetal insulin response to glucose infusion during fed state; results of five infusions in four animals. B. Fetal insulin response to glucose infusion during fasting state; results of three infusions in three animals. Mean ± 1 SD (bars) are given (61).

species. For example, in the rabbit, maternal weight does not increase significantly with pregnancy, and both the absolute and weight-specific maternal glucose turnover rates were not different in pregnant versus nonpregnant animals. By contrast, in guinea pigs, a species that usually carries a large fetal mass to term, the maternal glucose turnover rate per kilogram increases markedly when the conceptuses represent a relatively large percentage of the mother's weight, whereas the glucose turnover

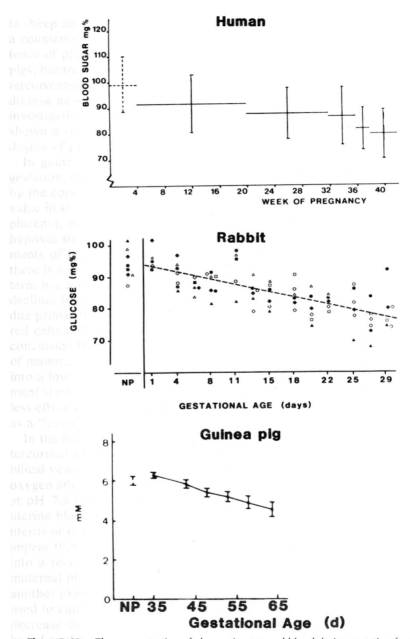

Figure 3-13: The concentration of glucose in maternal blood during gestation for humans (85), rabbits (27), and guinea pigs (76). NP, nonpregnant.

Table 3-12

**Comparison among Species of the Nonpregnant
versus Pregnant Animals Glucose Disposal Rates**

Species	Gestational age (days)	Glucose disposal rate (mg/kg/min)		Reference
		Nonpregnant	Pregnant	
Man	Term	2.43 ± 0.61	2.42 ± 0.51	48
Sheep	Term	2.00 ± 0.12	2.07 ± 0.21	40
Guinea pig	33–63	10.1 ± 1.3	12.1 ± 0.4	26
Rabbit	7–30	4.5 ± 0.4	3.7 ± 0.3	35
Rat[a]	21	9.4 ± 0.4	9.7 ± 0.5	53

[a] Not under chronic, steady-state conditions.

rate per kilogram is not significantly different from nonpregnant animals when there is only a single fetus representing approximately 10% of her weight (Figure 3-14) (29). Furthermore, there is a suppression of maternal glucose utilization rate during fasting, the degree of which is a function of total fetal mass. Thus, the impact of pregnancy upon the weight specific utilization rate in the mother is a function of several factors:

1. glucose utilization rate of the maternal nonuterine tissues;
2. glucose utilization rate of the uteroplacental tissues and of the fetus;
3. the relative proportion of total conceptus weight to total maternal weight;
4. the stage of gestation; and
5. the nutritional state of the mother.

Since the weight-specific glucose turnover rate is either constant or increasing during pregnancy and the maternal glucose concentration is falling, the calculated glucose clearance of the mother increases in all species studied (35). However, the interpretation of this change in glucose clearance induced by pregnancy is far from clear, and its physiologic meaning is more difficult to define than the changes in glucose turnover rate. It is interesting that the increased glucose clearance that occurs during pregnancy takes place despite a relative insulin resistance which develops during pregnancy and despite a tendency toward a diabetogenic state which also characterizes pregnancy. These apparently conflicting observations regarding glucose metabolism in the mother can be reconciled if the enlarging uterus and conceptus represent a site whose glucose consumption is not regulated by changes in maternal insulin concentration, that is, a noninsulin-dependent tissue mass in the mother. As we

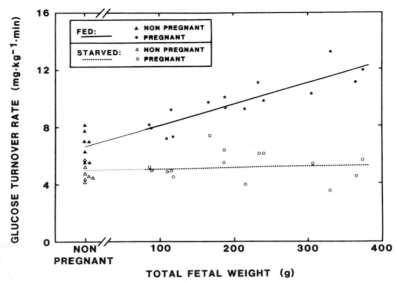

Figure 3-14: The relationship of glucose turnover rate to fetal mass in pregnant guinea pigs. The variability in fetal mass reflects differences in litter size among animals. Regression line for fed state values: glucose turnover rate (GTR) = (0.0143)(fetal mass) + 6.81, r = 0.9. Regression line for fasted state values: GTR = 0.001(fetal mass) + 5.0, r = 0.17. Reproduced from Gilbert *et al.* (29) by permission of S. Karger AG, Basel.

have seen, there is some evidence to support this interpretation, although the question is far from resolved.

Partition of Glucose between Mother and Conceptus

The previous discussion centered around the rate of turnover of maternal glucose without attempting to fractionate it into glucose consumed by the pregnant uterus and conceptus versus glucose used by the nonuterine tissues of the mother. The earliest attempt to describe the two components of maternal glucose turnover was made by Bergman (12) who compared glucose turnover rate in twin pregnant and nonpregnant sheep, as well as in lactating sheep (13). He found that if all of the differences were attributed to the pregnant uterus, this organ would account for approximately 20–40% of the maternal glucose turnover rate. This study design, of necessity, compares different groups of animals and makes the assumption that the glucose utilization by nonuterine tissues of the mother is comparable to that of the nonpregnant animal. Thus far, there has been only one study in which both maternal glucose turnover and glucose

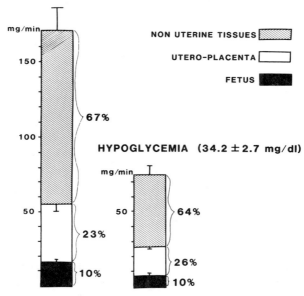

Figure 3-15: The partition of maternal glucose utilization in late gestation pregnant ewes in the fed and fasted states. While the absolute rates of utilization decrease in all three compartments, the partition among compartments stays constant; that is, there is no evidence of a sparing or protective effect on the uterus or fetus as glucose production rate in the mother decreases (34).

uptake by the uteroplacenta and the fetus have been measured in the same animal (34). Figure 3-15 taken from that report illustrates that in singleton pregnant sheep, approximately one-third of the glucose utilization of the mother is accounted for by the uterus, supporting the indirect evidence Bergman (12) had presented in twin pregnancy. Furthermore, Figure 3-15 demonstrates that maternal fasting does not alter markedly this relationship.

In other species we are just beginning to be provided with data for such calculations, and thus far, the two sets of data—uterine and maternal glucose utilization rates—have not been collected simultaneously in the same animals. Thus, current estimates of the percentage of maternal glucose utilization that can be attributed to the uterus and its contents must be regarded as fairly crude approximations. It is clear that in all the species that have been investigated, the uterus represents a major site of glucose utilization. The glucose requirements by the human pregnant uterus are likely to be high, reflecting the relatively large brain : body weight ratio of the human fetus and a placenta that is more permeable to glucose than that of some other species.

FRUCTOSE METABOLISM

Fructose is a six carbon sugar with a ketone group on the C_2 position and in this respect is different from the other two hexoses of importance in fetal and neonatal metabolism, glucose and galactose, which are both aldoses. Interest in the fetal metabolism of fructose stems primarily from the observation that in some species (e.g., sheep) the plasma concentration of fructose is very high throughout prenatal life and decreases rapidly after birth.

Huggett *et al.* (45) concluded from acute studies in pregnant sheep that the fructose in fetal blood originated in the placenta. From *in vitro* studies of Hers (41) on the sheep placenta and those of Alexander *et al.* (1) on the perfused sheep placenta *in situ,* it seems likely that fructose is produced from glucose through the intermediate formation of sorbitol, the straight chain alcohol derived from the reduction of glucose. The production of fructose by the placenta even in those species with high concentrations of fructose in fetal blood, such as the sheep and cow, must be at a low rate since no studies have been able to demonstrate any significant umbilical arteriovenous difference of fructose. This also implies that its rate of utilization by the fetus is relatively low.

A low rate of fructose utilization is strongly suggested by the studies of Warnes *et al.* (6, 86, 87) who found a very low clearance rate after a bolus injection of [^{14}C]fructose into the fetal lamb. The turnover rate of fructose they calculated from the bolus injection would represent approximately 0.12 mg/kg/min of fructose compared to the glucose utilization rate we reported of approximately 4–5 mg/kg/min. The fructose space calculated by Warnes *et al.* (86) was approximately equal to that of fetal extracellular fluid, which is 30% of the body weight. The methods they used, however, would tend to overestimate carbohydrate space in the fetus since their study did not attempt to correct for net tracer fluxes into the uteroplacental compartment from the fetus. We do not know the magnitude of this flux for fructose, although as pointed out earlier, the net uteroplacental tracer flux for glucose can be equal to approximately half of the infusion rate of glucose. Alexander *et al.* (1) in studies on an isolated perfused fetus also found little metabolism of [^{14}C]fructose in the fetal lamb and a low turnover rate. They noted that $^{14}CO_2$ derived from fructose increased as the glucose concentration decreased. These observations are consistent with our studies in fasted sheep under unstressed conditions, which found that as the glucose concentration in the mother and in the fetus fall during a maternal fast, fructose concentration in the fetus decreases slowly over several days suggesting some utilization of a fructose pool under these conditions. Dawes and Shelley (23) concluded that the rapid decline in fructose concentration that occurs after delivery was largely a function of renal excretion rather than metabolism. Thus, the role of the high fructose concentrations in fetal blood of some species is still unknown, but it would appear that one role is to act as a energy store that can be mobilized over some days under conditions of maternal fasting.

GALACTOSE METABOLISM

Galactose plays only a small role in fetal metabolism but a very important role in neonatal metabolism. Perhaps because of the importance of its neonatal role, it is not surprising that the fetal liver is already prepared to handle the metabolism of fairly large galactose loads. Galactose is phosphorylated in the liver by galactokinase and then through a series of reactions is converted to glucose. In the rat, rhesus monkey, and human fetuses the enzymes required for galactose metabolism are present in fetal liver well before birth. In fact, in the monkey the enzyme activity of the three enzymes specific for galactose metabolism are higher in fetal life than they are postnatally, although the metabolic capacity of the liver for metabolizing galactose is greater in the neonate (72). This is one example where changes in enzyme activity can be misleading, presumably because the activity is not rate limiting even in the neonatal period.

The placenta of the rat is the only placental type that has been studied with regard to galactose permeability. Several studies have shown that when galactose is elevated in maternal blood by dietary manipulation, it is increased in fetal blood to a level approximately equal to that of the mother (67). However, under normal circumstances there is very little galactose present in maternal and/or fetal blood. Therefore, galactose is of little importance nutritionally to the fetus. In sharp contrast, once the fetus is delivered it is suddenly presented with a diet in which galactose plays a major role, since lactose, which is a disaccharide composed of glucose and galactose, is the principal carbohydrate in the milk of mammals. Thus, glucose and galactose are presented to the newborn in equal amounts. At the concentrations of lactose in human milk, an infant receives 3.4 g of galactose per 100 ml of milk, which is far more than any other glucogenic precursor. Galactose concentration in the blood of newborn infants is very low because of a remarkable rate of hepatic uptake and utilization. In studies of the perfused fetal liver of the rhesus monkey

(71), it was found that galactose was rapidly taken up by the liver in contrast to glucose, and its uptake was independent of insulin concentration. Furthermore, a net increase in liver glycogen was only achieved when galactose was present in the perfusate. In human newborn infants, galactose clearance is very rapid compared to that of glucose, 6.9% disappearance per minute versus 1.4% per minute (8). Thus, its role appears to be that of a carbohydrate that can be present in the diet in large amounts without stimulating hyperinsulinemia, can be rapidly cleared by the liver leading to net glycogen accumulation, and finally, may play an important role in glycogen regulation within the neonatal liver.

From a comparative viewpoint, it is of interest that some mammals produce milk with very low or absent lactose content. These include the aquatic mammals; for example, the California sea lion (55) and some marsupials (84) produce milk completely free of lactose (55). The low lactose content of kangaroo milk is associated with low levels of intestinal lactase (50) and a deficiency of galactokinase and galactose-1-phosphate uridyl transferase (81). Thus, in some mammalian newborns galactose metabolism will play a far less significant role than it does in humans and other mammals with high lactose concentrations in the breast milk.

LACTATE METABOLISM

After glucose, lactate represents the major carbohydrate consumed by the mammalian fetus. Historically, it also represents a substrate whose metabolism has been misinterpreted by perinatal physiologists. We shall review the evidence supporting the conclusion that lactate is an important fetal nutrient which is used as a fuel and carbon source for growth.

Lactate concentrations have been shown to be higher in fetal blood compared to maternal blood in many different species including humans. This was probably first demonstrated by Eastman and McLane in 1931 (24). In the following years it was well established that fetal arterial blood has a much lower oxygen tension than that of postnatal life (see Chapter 6). Understandably, the higher lactate concentration in fetal blood was interpreted as reflecting a chronic state of hypoxia in the fetus, the concept of the fetal environment representing "Mount Everest *in utero*." The metabolic implication was that the fetus is a net producer of lactate and that a high rate of fetal lactate production is the reason for the high lactate concentrations in fetal blood. It was presumed that lactate, as an end-product of anaerobic metabolism, was being excreted out of the umbilical circulation into the placenta, much as the fetus excretes metabolic end products such as urea and carbon dioxide. Attempts to establish this hypothesis were plagued by the lack of techniques for studying animals under conscious, unstressed conditions. For example, Huckabee *et al.* (44) in 1962 reported lactate and pyruvate concentrations across the uterine and umbilical circulations of pregnant goats. The animals were studied while under light anesthesia and immediately after the catheters were placed. These investigators were unable to show any consistent pattern to the uterine and umbilical arteriovenous differences. In fact, a very wide range of both negative and positive arteriovenous differences were found.

Ample evidence has been collected for humans that demonstrates the presence of a metabolic acidosis in cord blood secondary to a lactic acidemia under conditions of perinatal asphyxia. Stembera and Hodr (80) demonstrated a significant positive arteriovenous difference for lactate across the umbilical circulation under conditions of perinatal asphyxia. Under those conditions the fetus clearly is a net producer of lactate, which is then excreted into the placenta. Since then numerous clinical publications have confirmed that the umbilical arteriovenous difference of lactate is frequently positive. These observations should not be interpreted as reflecting a pattern of metabolism in the fetus as it develops *in utero* and prior to the onset of labor. The conditions under which the clinical studies are carried out are very different from normal conditions *in utero* during the period of gestation preceding labor. We know that under normal physiologic conditions, the low oxygen tension in fetal blood does not represent an inadequate oxygen supply (see Chapter 6). Tissues of the fetus in humans and other animals are adequately oxygenated. The acid base pattern in fetal blood during most of the pregnancy excluding parturition is that of a mild compensated respiratory acidosis rather than a pattern of metabolic acidosis. What then is the role of lactate in fetal metabolism throughout pregnancy excluding the time of parturition?

The first clue to answering this question came from data describing persistently higher lactate concentrations in the umbilical vein compared to the umbilical artery in the fetal lamb studied under conscious, unstressed, steady-state conditions during the last 20% of gestation (18). These data clearly demonstrated that the fetus is a net consumer of lactate under normal conditions and that the quantity of lactate received from the placenta is appreciable, representing approximately 25% of the oxygen consumption if all the lactate was oxidized. This same study demonstrated a similar venous–arterial lactate difference in the uterine circulation, establishing the fact that the intervening tissues between the umbilical and uterine circulations, what we have called the *uteroplacenta,* are producing lactate and releasing it into both circulations. Figure 3-16 presents more recent data in which the concentration of lactate in fetal arterial blood is set equal to 100 and the concentrations in the other three

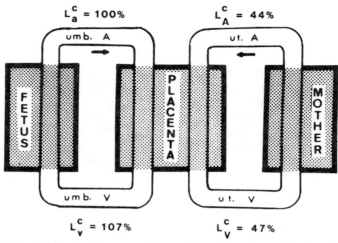

Figure 3-16: Relative lactate concentration relationships in the umbilical and uterine circulations of chronically catheterized sheep. Concentrations are expressed as the percentage of the concentration in the fetal artery which is set at 100% (77). Reproduced from *The Journal of Clinical Investigation*, 1982, **70**, 179–192, by copyright permission of The American Society for Clinical Investigation.

vessels are presented as a percentage of the fetal arterial concentration (77).

The uterine lactate/oxygen quotients have been measured in several species besides the sheep, all studied under chronic, steady-state conditions (Table 3-13). It is clear that lactate is released from the pregnant uterus into the maternal circulation in all species studied thus far. In the cow and sheep, where umbilical uptakes have been measured, lactate is released from the uteroplacental tissues into the umbilical circulation as well. It is an interesting and unresolved question at this time why the placenta produces lactate from glucose under aerobic conditions and what, if any, advantage lactate has as a fetal nutrient over glucose. The release of lactate from the uteroplacental tissues does not follow simple concentration differences in that in late gestation a larger quantity of lactate is delivered into the fetal circulation than into the maternal circulation despite a higher lactate concentration in the fetus (21, 78). Moll *et al.* (59) have presented data collected from *in vitro* studies of the perfused guinea pig placenta that suggest that there may be a carrier system in the placenta for lactate. However, this is not yet clear since little stereospecificity was demonstrated in those studies. Similar evidence suggesting a specific lactate carrier system within the placenta has been obtained by Carstensen *et al.* for the *in vitro* perfused human placenta (20). The pla-

Table 3-13

Glucose and Lactate Oxygen Quotients across the Uterine Circulation in Several Species

Species	Gestational age (days)	Oxygen quotients			Reference
		Glucose	Lactate	Glucose + lactate	
Sheep	120–145	0.80	−0.08	+0.72	57
	71–81	0.76	−0.16	+0.60	
Cow	Late gestation	0.83			21
Horse	Late gestation	0.96			69
Guinea pig	40–49	1.22	−0.47	+0.75	15
	50–63	1.26	−0.47	+0.79	16
Rabbit	20–30	1.50	−0.90	+0.60	46
	24	1.70	−0.83	+0.87	46
	30	2.30	−1.12	+1.18	28

cental supply of lactate to the fetus is substantial (in the fetal lamb it is approximately 2 mg/kg/min). This rate exceeds the net consumption of any other carbon compound other than glucose.

Fetal Lactate Utilization

Fetal lactate utilization can be determined by the same approach employed for glucose utilization, that is, by the infusion of tracer lactate into the fetal circulation (77). The net tracer flux from the fetal compartment into the uteroplacental compartment is much less for lactate than for glucose. During an infusion of [U-^{14}C]lactate into the fetal lamb, the net tracer lactate loss into the placenta represented only 8.0 ± 1.0% of the rate of infusion, in contrast to the 53% loss during a [^{14}C]glucose infusion. Having determined the net tracer lactate loss from the fetal compartment, fetal lactate utilization can be calculated. Lactate utilization in the fetal lamb in the last 20% of gestation is three times higher than the umbilical uptake with a mean value of 5.9 ± 0.7 mg/kg/min, compared to an umbilical uptake of 1.95 ± 0.16 mg/kg/min. Thus, there is a fairly high rate of lactate production (approximately 4 mg/kg/min) even in the normal well-oxygenated fetus. Within the fetus, some organs are net lactate producers and some are net lactate consumers. Studies of net substrate flow across the fetal hind limb have established that the carcass is at least one of the sites of net lactate production. At one time it was believed that the fetal brain produced large quantities of lactate, but that hypothesis was based entirely upon *in vitro* experimental studies. *In vivo* studies of fetal cere-

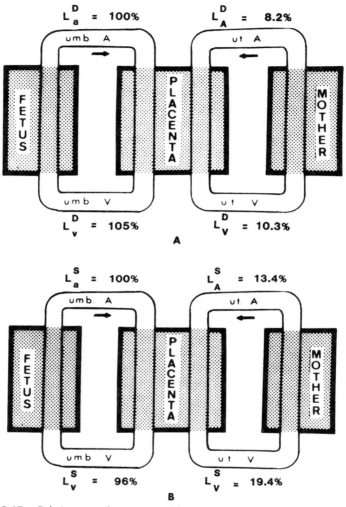

Figure 3-17: Relative tracer lactate (A) and lactate specific activity (B) relationships in the umbilical and uterine circulations of chronically catheterized sheep, during infusion of [U-^{14}C]glucose into the fetal circulation. Concentrations are expressed as the percentage of the concentration in the fetal artery, which is set at 100%. Drawn from data by Ref. 77.

bral metabolism have not shown a large efflux of lactate from the cerebral circulation (47).

Net lactate consumption has been described for the fetal heart, but this organ is a relatively small percentage of total body weight, and thus its lactate uptake would represent a small part of total fetal lactate utilization. Fisher *et al.* (25) reported a net lactate uptake by the fetal heart of

73 $\mu M/100$ g/min at 120 days gestation which for an organ weighing 15 g would represent a lactate utilization of 11 μM/min. This is only 13% of the total lactate utilization described by Sparks *et al.* (77) for the fetus as a whole. Preliminary studies by Sparks *et al.* suggest that the fetal liver is a major site of lactate utilization, although as pointed out earlier, only a small fraction of this lactate utilization can be accounted for by glucogenesis.

During an infusion of [^{14}C]glucose into the fetus, fetal lactate production from glucose can be estimated. Figure 3-17A presents the tracer lactate concentration relationships in the same format as the lactate concentrations presented in Figure 3-16. During the tracer glucose infusion into the fetus, the umbilical venous tracer lactate concentration was consistently 5% higher than that in the umbilical artery, thus establishing that the uteroplacenta must have produced lactate from labeled fetal glucose. Figure 3-17B presents the same relationships for lactate-specific activity. In this case the umbilical vein has a lower specific activity than the umbilical artery, despite the higher tracer concentrations, reflecting the production of unlabeled lactate from maternal glucose within the placenta. Since umbilical blood increases its specific activity as it perfuses the fetus, the specific activity relationships establish that the fetus is producing labeled lactate from labeled glucose.

Taken together, Figures 3-16 and 3-17 illustrate the importance of separately analyzing tracer and tracee concentrations as well as specific activity relationships within the fetus. Each analysis demonstrates a different aspect of lactate metabolism, information that would have been lost by confining the analysis to specific activity relationships alone.

Figure 3-18 summarizes current information about the lactate fluxes

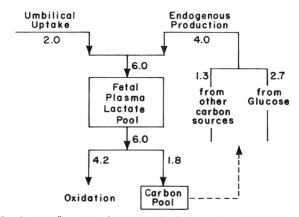

Figure 3-18: Lactate fluxes (mg/kg/min) in the late gestation fetal lamb determined in our laboratories in a series of studies (18, 33, 77).

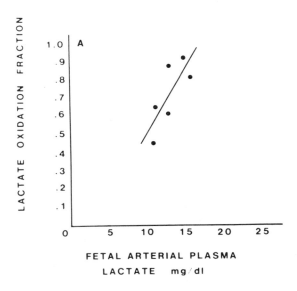

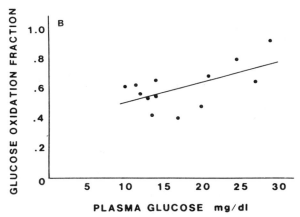

Figure 3-19: Lactate (A) and glucose (B) oxidation fractions for late gestation fetal lambs. Lactate data obtained for 6 fetuses infused with [U-14C]lactate; glucose data obtained for 13 fetuses infused with [U-14C]glucose (33).

into and out of the fetal plasma lactate pool (77). The fetal lactate oxidation rate has been estimated to represent approximately 70% of the fetal lactate utilization rate or approximately 4 mg/kg/min (33). The rest of the lactate enters the carbon pool either as carbon accretion or in carbon recycling. If one sums the oxidation rates of glucose and lactate in the fetal lamb after correction for the interconversion of glucose and lactate, both rates account for approximately 0.16 mmol/kg/min of oxygen, or approximately 50% of fetal oxygen consumption.

There is some evidence suggesting a carbohydrate sparing effect on fetal metabolism as shown in Figures 3-19A and B (33), which presents the fractional lactate oxidation rates and fractional glucose oxidation rates as a function of their respective concentrations. The figure demonstrates that as their concentrations in the blood increase, the fractional oxidation rates of glucose and lactate increase. Since fetal oxygen consumption is not altered, it is clear that the oxidation of carbohydrates spares the oxidation of other substrates. Conversely, as glucose and lactate concentrations fall, the oxidation of alternate fuels increases. We suspect that the other substrates most involved are amino acids for reasons discussed in Chapter 4.

REFERENCES

1. Alexander, D.P., Britton, H.G. and Nixon, D.A. (1970). *The metabolism of fructose and glucose by the sheep foetus: Studies on the isolated perfused preparation with radioactively labelled sugars.* Quarterly Journal of Experimental Physiology **55**, 346–362.
2. Anand, R.S., Ganguli, S. and Sperling, M.A. (1980). *Effect of insulin-induced maternal hypoglycemia on glucose turnover in maternal and fetal sheep.* American Journal of Physiology **238**, E524–E532.
3. Bassett, J.J. and Madill, D. (1974). *Influence of prolonged glucose infusions on plasma insulin and growth hormone concentrations of foetal lambs.* Journal of Endocrinology **62**, 299–309.
4. Battaglia, F.C. (1978). *Commonality and diversity in fetal development: Bridging the interspecies gap.* Pediatric Research **12**, 736–745.
5. Battaglia, F.C. and Hay, W.W. Jr. (1984). *Energy and substrate requirements for fetal and placental growth and metabolism. In* "Fetal Physiology and Medicine" (R.W. Beard and P.W. Nathanielsz, eds.), pp 601–628, Marcel Dekker Publications, New York.
6. Battaglia, F.C. and Meschia, G. (1978). *Principal substrates of fetal metabolism.* Physiologic Reviews **58**, 499–527.
7. Battaglia, F.C. and Meschia, G. (1981). *Fetal and placental metabolisms: Their interrelationship and impact upon maternal metabolism.* Proceedings of the Nutrition Society **40**, 99–113.
8. Battaglia, F.C. and Sparks, J.W. (1983). *Perinatal nutrition and metabolism. In* "Pediatrics 2: Perinatal Medicine" (R.D.H. Boyd and F.C. Battaglia, eds.), pp 145–171, Butterworths, London.
9. Behrman, R.E., Lees, M.H., Peterson, E.N., DeLannoy, C.W. and Seeds, A.E. (1970). *Distribution of the circulation in the normal and asphyxiated fetal primate.* American Journal of Obstetrics and Gynecology **108**, 956–969.
10. Bell, A.W., Battaglia, F.C., Makowski, E.L. and Meschia, G. (1985). *Relationship between metabolic rate and body size in fetal life.* Biology of the Neonate **47**, 120–123.
11. Bell, A.W., Kennaugh, J.M., Battaglia, F.C., Makowski, E.L. and Meschia, G. (1986). *Metabolic and circulatory studies of the fetal lamb at mid gestation.* American Journal of Physiology **250**, E538–E544.

12. Bergman, E.N. (1963). *Quantitative aspects of glucose metabolism in pregnant and non-pregnant sheep*. American Journal of Physiology **204**, 147–152.
13. Bergman, E.N. and Hogue, D.E. (1967). *Glucose turnover and oxidation rates in lactating sheep*. American Journal of Physiology **213**, 1378–1384.
14. Blazquez, E., Lipshaw, L.A., Blazquez, M. and Foa, P.P. (1975). *The synthesis and release of insulin in fetal, nursing, and young adult rats: studies in vivo and in vitro*. Pediatric Research **9**, 17–25.
15. Block, S.M., Sparks, J.W., Johnson, R.L. and Battaglia, F.C. (1985). *Metabolic quotients of the gravid uterus of the chronically catheterized guinea pig*. Pediatric Research **19**, 840–845.
16. Block, S.M., Johnson, R.L., Sparks, J.W. and Battaglia, F.C. (In preparation). *Uterine metabolism of the pregnant guinea pig as a function of gestational age*.
17. Bohr, C. (1900). *Der respiratorische stoffwechsel des sauge-thierembryo*. Skandinavia Archives of Physiology **15**, 413–424.
18. Burd, L.I., Jones, M.D. Jr., Simmons, M.A., Makowski, E.L., Meschia, G. and Battaglia, F.C. (1975). *Placental production and foetal utilization of lactate and pyruvate*. Nature **254**, 210–211.
19. Carson, B.S., Philipps, A.F., Simmons, M.A., Battaglia, F.C. and Meschia, G. (1980). *Effects of a sustained insulin infusion upon glucose uptake and oxygenation of the ovine fetus*. Pediatric Research **14**, 147–152.
20. Carstensen, M.H., Leichtweiss, H.-P. and Schroder, H. (1983). *Lactate carriers in the artificially perfused human term placenta*. Placenta **4**, 165–174.
20a. Chinard, F.P., Danesino, V., Hartman, W.L., Huggett, A. St.G., Paul, W. and Reynolds, S.R.M. (1956). *The transmission of hexoses across the placenta in the human and the rhesus monkey*. Journal of Physiology **132**, 289–303.
20b. Coltart, T.M., Beard, R.W., Turner, R.C. and Oakley, N.W. (1969). *Blood glucose and insulin relationships in the human mother and fetus before onset of labor*. British Medical Journal **4**, 17–19.
21. Comline, R.S. and Silver, M. (1976). *Some aspects of foetal and utero-placental metabolism in cows with indwelling umbilical and uterine vascular catheters*. Journal of Physiology **260**, 571–586.
22. Cross, K.W. (1979). *La Chaleur Animale and the infant brain*. Journal of Physiology **294**, 1–21.
23. Dawes G.S. and Shelley, H.J. (1962). *Fate of glucose in newly delivered foetal lambs*. Nature **194**, 296–297.
24. Eastman, N.J. and McLane, C.M. (1931). *The lactic acid content of umbilical cord blood under various conditions*. Bulletin of Johns Hopkins Hospital **48**, 261–268.
25. Fisher, D.J., Heymann, M.A. and Rudolph, A.M. (1980). *Myocardial oxygen and carbohydrate consumption in fetal lambs in utero and in adult sheep*. American Journal of Physiology **238**, H399–H405.
26. Gilbert, M., Sparks, J.W., Girard, J. and Battaglia, F.C. (1982). *Glucose turnover rate during pregnancy in the conscious guinea pig*. Pediatric Research **16**, 310–313.
27. Gilbert, M., Hay, W.W. Jr., Johnson, R.L. and Battaglia, F.C. (1984). *Some aspects of maternal metabolism throughout pregnancy in the conscious rabbit*. Pediatric Research **18**, 854–859.
28. Gilbert, M., Hauguel, S. and Bouisset, M. (1984). *Uterine blood flow and substrate uptake in conscious rabbit during late gestation*. American Journal of Physiology **247**, E574–E580.
29. Gilbert, M., Sparks, J.W. and Battaglia, F.C. (1985). *Effects of fasting on glucose turnover and metabolite levels in conscious, pregnant guinea pigs*. Biology of the Neonate **48**, 85–89.

30. Girard, J.R., Ferre, P., Gilbert, M., Kervran, A., Assan, R. and Marliss, E.B. (1977). *Foetal metabolic response to maternal fasting in the rat.* American Journal of Physiology **232**, E456–E463.
31. Goodner, C.J. and Thompson, D.J. (1967). *Glucose metabolism in the fetus in utero: The effect of maternal fasting and glucose loading in the rat.* Pediatric Research **1**, 443–451.
32. Hay, W.W. Jr., Sparks, J.W., Quissell, B., Battaglia, F.C. and Meschia, G. (1981). *Simultaneous measurements of umbilical uptake, fetal utilization rate and fetal turnover rate of glucose.* American Journal of Physiology **240**, E662–E668.
33. Hay, W.W. Jr., Myers, S.A., Sparks, J.W., Wilkening, R.W., Meschia, G. and Battaglia, F.C. (1983). *Glucose and lactate oxidation rates in the fetal lamb.* Proceedings of the Society for Experimental Biology and Medicine **173**, 553–563.
34. Hay, W.W. Jr., Sparks, J.W., Wilkening, R.B., Battaglia, F.C. and Meschia, G. (1983). *Partition of maternal glucose production between conceptus and maternal tissues in sheep.* American Journal of Physiology **245**, E347–E350.
35. Hay, W.W. Jr., Gilbert, M., Johnson, R.L. and Battaglia, F.C. (1984). *Glucose turnover rates in chronically catheterized non-pregnant and pregnant rabbits.* Pediatric Research **18**, 276–280.
36. Hay, W.W. Jr., Sparks, J.W., Battaglia, F.C. and Meschia, G. (1984). *Maternal-fetal glucose exchange: Necessity of a 3 pool model.* American Journal of Physiology **246**, E528–E534.
37. Hay, W.W. Jr., Sparks, J.W., Gilbert, M., Battaglia, F.C. and Meschia, G. (1984). *Effect of insulin on glucose uptake by the maternal hindlimb and uterus and by the fetus in conscious pregnant sheep.* Journal of Endocrinology **100**, 119–124.
38. Hay, W.W. Jr., Sparks, J.W., Wilkening, R.B., Battaglia, F.C. and Meschia, G. (1984). *Fetal glucose uptake and utilization as functions of maternal glucose concentration.* American Journal of Physiology **246**, E237–E242.
39. Hay, W.W. Jr., Meznarich, H.K., Sparks, J.W., Battaglia, F.C. and Meschia, G. (1985). *Effect of insulin on glucose uptake in near-term fetal lambs (42042).* Proceedings of the Society for Experimental Biology and Medicine **178**, 557–564.
40. Hay, W.W. Jr., Lin, C.-C., Meznarich, H.K. and Battaglia, F.C. (In preparation). *Insulin sensitivity of uterine and non-uterine tissues of the pregnant sheep.*
41. Hers, H.G. (1960). *Le mecanisme de la formation du fructose seminal et du fructose foetal.* Biochimica Biophysica Acta **37**, 127–138.
42. Hodgson, J.C., Mellor, D.J. and Field, A.C. (1980). *Rates of glucose production and utilization by the foetus in chronically catheterized sheep.* Biochemical Journal **186**, 739–747.
43. Holzman, I.R., Lemons, J.A., Meschia, G. and Battaglia, F.C. (1979). *Uterine uptake of amino acids and glutamine-glutamate balance across the placenta of the pregnant ewe.* Journal of Developmental Physiology **1**, 137–149.
44. Huckabee, W.E., Metcalfe, J., Prystowsky, H. and Barron, D.H. (1962). *Movements of lactate and pyruvate in pregnant uterus.* American Journal of Physiology **202**, 193–197.
45. Huggett, A.St.G., Warren, F.L. and Warren, N.V. (1951). *The origin of the blood fructose of the foetal sheep.* Journal of Physiology **113**, 258–275.
46. Johnson, R.L., Gilbert, M., Block, S.M. and Battaglia, F.C. (1986). *Uterine metabolism of the pregnant rabbit under chronic steady-state conditions.* American Journal of Obstetrics and Gynecology **154**, 1146–1151.
47. Jones, M.D. Jr., Burd, L.I., Makowski, E.L., Meschia, G. and Battaglia, F.C. (1975). *Cerebral metabolism in sheep: a comparative study of the adult, the lamb, and the fetus.* American Journal of Physiology **229**, 235–239.
48. Kalhan, S.C., D'Angelo, L.J., Savin, S.M. and Adam, P.A.J. (1979). *Glucose produc-

tion in pregnant women at term gestation. Journal of Clinical Investigation **63**, 388–394.

49. Katz, J. (1982). *Importance of sites of tracer administration and sampling in turnover studies*. Federation Proceedings **41**, 123–128.
50. Kerry, K.R. (1969). *Intestinal disaccharidase activity in a monotreme and eight species of marsupials (with an added note on the disaccharidases of five species of sea birds)*. Comprehensive Biochemical Physiology **29**, 1015–1022.
51. Kleiber, M. (1975) "The Fire of Life. An Introduction to Animal Energetics," Robert E. Krieger Publishing Company, Huntington, New York.
52. Leitch, I., Hytten, F.E. and Billewicz, W.Z. (1959). *The maternal and neonatal weights of some mammalia*. Proceedings of the Zoological Society, London **133**, 11–29.
53. Leturque, A., Gilbert, M. and Girard, J. (1981). *Glucose turnover during pregnancy in anaesthetized post-absorptive rats*. Biochemical Journal **196**, 633–636.
54. Leutenegger, W. (1972). *Newborn size and pelvic dimensions of australopithecus*. Nature **240**, 568–569.
55. Mathai, C.K., Pilson, M.E.Q. and Buetler, E. (1966). *Galactose metabolism in the sea lion*. Proceedings of the Society for Experimental Biology and Medicine **123**, 603–604.
56. Meier, P.R., Manchester, D.K., Battaglia, F.C. and Meschia, G. (1983). *Fetal heart rate in relation to body mass*. Proceedings of the Society for Experimental Biology and Medicine **172**, 107–110.
57. Meschia, G., Battaglia, F.C., Hay, W.W. Jr. and Sparks, J.W. (1980). *Utilization of substrates by the ovine placenta in vivo*. Federation Proceedings **39**, 245–249.
58. Moll, W., Kunzel, W. and Ross, H.G. (1970). *Gas exchange of the pregnant uterus of anesthetized and unanesthetized guinea pigs*. Respiratory Physiology **8**, 303–318.
59. Moll, W., Girard, H. and Gros, G. (1980). *Facilitated diffusion of lactic acid in the guinea-pig placenta*. Pflugers Archives **385**, 229–238.
60. Morriss, F.H. Jr., Makowski, E.L., Meschia, G. and Battaglia, F.C. (1975). *The glucose/oxygen quotient of the term human fetus*. Biology of the Neonate **25**, 44–52.
61. Philipps, A.F., Carson, B.S., Meschia, G. and Battaglia, F.C. (1978). *Insulin secretion in fetal and newborn sheep*. American Journal of Physiology **235**, E467–E474.
62. Prior, R.L. (1982). *Gluconeogenesis in the ruminant fetus: Evaluation of conflicting evidence from radiotracer and other experimental techniques*. Federation Proceedings **41**, 117–122.
63. Prior, R.L. and Christenson, R.K. (1977). *Gluconeogenesis from alanine in vivo by the ovine fetus and lamb*. American Journal of Physiology **233**, E462–E468.
64. Riggs, D.S. (1963). "The Mathematical Approach to Physiological Problems," Williams and Wilkins Company, Baltimore.
65. Sandiford, I. and Wheeler, T. (1924). *The basal metabolism before, during and after pregnancy*. Journal of Biologic Chemistry **62**, 329–350.
66. Schroder, H., Leichtweiss, H.P. and Madee, W. (1975). *The transport of D-glucose, L-glucose and D-mannose across the isolated guinea pig placenta*. Pflugers Archives **356**, 267–275.
67. Segal, S. and Bernstein, H. (1963). *Observations on cataract formation in newborn offsprings of cats fed a high-galactose diet*. Journal of Pediatrics **62**, 363–370.
68. Shelley, H.J. (1961). *Glycogen reserves and their changes at birth*. British Medical Bulletin **17**, 137–143.
69. Silver, M. and Comline, R.S. (1976). *Fetal and placental O_2 consumption and the uptake of different metabolites in the ruminant and horse during late gestation*. *In* "Oxygen Transport to Tissue II—Advances in Experimental Medicine and Biology," (D.D. Reneau and J. Grote, eds.), Volume 75, pp 731–736, Plenum, New York.

70. Silver, M., Steven, D.H. and Comline, R.S. (1973). *Placental exchange and morphology in ruminants and mare. In* "Foetal and Neonatal Physiology, Barcroft Centenary Symposium," (R.S. Comline, K.W. Cross, G.S. Dawes and P.W. Nathanielsz, eds.), pp 245–271, Cambridge University Press, London.

71. Sparks, J.W., Lynch, A., Chez, R.A. and Glinsmann, W.H. (1976). *Glycogen regulation in isolated perfused near term monkey liver.* Pediatric Research **10**, 51–56.

72. Sparks, J.W., Lynch, A. and Glinsmann, W.H. (1976). *Regulation of rat liver glycogen synthesis and activities of glycogen cycle enzymes by glucose and galactose.* Metabolism **25**, 47–55.

73. Simmons, M.A., Jones, M.D. Jr., Battaglia, F.C. and Meschia, G. (1978). *Insulin effect on fetal glucose utilization.* Pediatric Research **12**, 90–92.

74. Simmons, M.A., Battaglia, F.C. and Meschia, G. (1979). *Placental transfer of glucose.* Journal of Developmental Physiology **1**, 227–243.

75. Sparks, J.W., Girard, J. and Battaglia, F.C. (1980). *An estimate of the caloric requirements of the human fetus.* Biology of the Neonate **38**, 113–119.

76. Sparks, J.W., Pegorier, J.-P., Girard, J. and Battaglia, F.C. (1981). *Substrate concentration changes during pregnancy in the guinea pig studied under unstressed steady state conditions.* Pediatric Research **15**, 1340–1344.

77. Sparks, J.W., Hay, W.W. Jr., Bonds, D., Meschia, G. and Battaglia, F.C. (1982). *Simultaneous measurements of lactate turnover rate and umbilical lactate uptake in the fetal lamb.* Journal of Clinical Investigation **70**, 179–192.

78. Sparks, J.W., Hay, W.W. Jr., Meschia, G. and Battaglia, F.C. (1983). *Partition of maternal nutrients to the placenta and fetus in the sheep.* European Journal of Obstetrics, Gynecology, and Reproductive Biology **14**, 331–340.

79. Stacey, T.E., Weedon, A.P., Haworth, C., Ward, R.H.T. and Boyd, R.D.H. (1978). *Fetomaternal transfer of glucose analogues by sheep placenta.* American Journal of Physiology **234**, E32–E37.

80. Stembera, Z.K. and Hodr, J. (1966). *I. The relationship between the blood levels of glucose, lactic acid and pyruvic acid in the mother and in both umbilical vessels of the healthy fetus.* Biology of the Neonate **10**, 227–238.

81. Stephens, T., Irvine, S., Mutton, P., Gupta, J.D. and Harley, J.D. (1974). *Deficiency of two enzymes of galactose metabolism in kangaroos.* Nature **248**, 524–525.

82. Thompson, G.E. and Bell, A.W. (1976). *Heat production in the newborn ox during noradrenaline infusion.* Biology of the Neonate **28**, 375–381.

83. Tsoulos, N.G., Colwill, J.R., Battaglia, F.C., Makowski, E.L. and Meschia, G. (1971). *Comparison of glucose, fructose and O_2 uptakes by fetuses of fed and starved ewes.* American Journal of Physiology **221**, 234–237.

84. Tyndale-Biscoe, H. (1973). "Life of Marsupials," Edward Arnold (Publishers) Limited, London.

85. Victor, A. (1974). *Normal blood sugar glucose variation during pregnancy.* Acta Obstetrica Gynecologia Scandanavia **53**, 37–40.

86. Warnes, D.M., Seamark, R.F. and Ballard, F.J. (1977). *Metabolism of glucose, fructose and lactate in vivo in chronically cannulated foetuses and in suckling lambs.* Biochemical Journal **162**, 617–626.

87. Warnes, D.M., Seamark, R.F. and Ballard, F.J. (1977). *The appearance of gluconeogenesis at birth in sheep.* Biochemical Journal **162**, 627–634.

88. Widdas, W.F. (1952). *Inability of diffusion to account for placental glucose transfer in the sheep and consideration of the kinetics of a possible carrier transfer.* Journal of Physiology **118**, 23–39.

89. Woods, L.L., Thornburg, K.L. and Faber, J.J. (1978). *Transplacental gradients in the guinea pig.* American Journal of Physiology **235**, H200–H207.

4

Fetal and Placental Metabolism:
Part II. Amino Acids and Lipids

NITROGEN AND AMINO ACID BALANCE IN THE FETUS

From measurements of nitrogen concentration in fetuses at different ages, the rate of nitrogen accretion within the fetus can be calculated. The nitrogen in the fetus can be divided into that contained in proteins and free amino acids versus that present in all other substances in the body including nucleic acids.

Where total amino acid concentrations in fetuses and newborns have been determined, the concentrations are similar among species at comparable stages of maturation (4, 38, 58, 60, 70). To facilitate calculation of total carbon and nitrogen accretion attributable to amino acid accretion, we have included Table 4-1 which lists the basic information required for each amino acid. The carbon:nitrogen ratio in individual amino acids varies from a maximum of 7.7 for the aromatic amino acids tyrosine and phenylalanine to a low of 1.28 for the basic amino acid arginine. The carbon:nitrogen ratio attributed to an "average" protein is 3.2. We cannot assume, however, that the carbon:nitrogen ratio of body protein remains constant during development when the proportion of collagen to total body protein is changing. For example, hydroxyproline and glycine concentrations increase with age as collagen increases in relation to other proteins (38). Because of the changing proportions of amino acids with

Table 4-1

Amino Acid Composition

Amino acid	Molecular weight	Number of carbon atoms	Number of nitrogen atoms	Percent carbon atoms	Percent nitrogen atoms	Carbon : nitrogen ratio
Essential amino acids						
Lys	146.19	6	2	49.25	19.15	2.57
His	155.16	5	3	38.67	27.07	1.43
Thr	119.12	4	1	40.29	11.75	3.43
Val	117.15	5	1	51.22	11.95	4.29
Met	149.22	5	1	40.21	9.38	4.29
I-Leu	131.18	6	1	54.89	10.67	5.14
Leu	131.18	6	1	54.89	10.67	5.14
Phe	165.19	9	1	65.39	8.48	7.71
Tryp	204.23	11	2	64.63	13.71	4.71
Nonessential amino acids						
Orn	132.16	5	2	45.40	21.19	2.14
Arg	174.21	6	4	41.33	32.14	1.28
Tau	125.15	2	1	19.18	11.19	1.71
Asp	133.10	4	1	36.06	10.52	3.43
Asn	150.14	4	2	31.97	18.65	1.71
Ser	105.09	3	1	34.26	13.32	2.57
Glu	147.13	5	1	40.78	9.52	4.28
Gln	146.15	5	2	41.05	19.16	2.14
Gly	75.07	2	1	31.97	18.65	1.71
Ala	89.09	3	1	40.41	15.71	2.57
Cys	121.15	3	1	29.71	11.56	2.57
Tyr	181.19	9	1	59.61	7.73	7.71
Pro	115.13	5	1	52.11	12.16	4.28
OH-Pro	131.13	5	1	45.76	10.68	4.28

different carbon : nitrogen ratios during development, the overall carbon : nitrogen ratio decreases in the fetal lamb from 3.42 at 66 days gestation to 3.06 at term.

When the total nitrogen versus total amino acid nitrogen in the fetus of the guinea pig (60) and the sheep (38) are compared, amino acid nitrogen represents approximately 81% of the total nitrogen in both species. Given this information, it would appear that a rough approximation of the rate of accretion of individual amino acids during growth could be obtained in any species from measurements of total nitrogen concentration during growth, assuming that 81% of this is amino acid nitrogen and that the proportion of individual amino acids to total nitrogen is similar to that presented in Table 4-2 for the fetal guinea pig and fetal lamb in late gestation.

Table 4-2

**Amino Acid Concentration
in Fetal Whole Body Homogenates**[a]

Amino acid	Guinea pigs 40–68 days gestation	Sheep 130–145 days gestation
Tau	0.22 ± 0.02	0.36 ± 0.03
Gly	6.44 ± 0.10	9.27 ± 0.44
Glu[b]	11.26 ± 0.29	11.42 ± 0.45
Ala	5.38 ± 0.10	6.18 ± 0.33
Ser	4.48 ± 0.12	4.12 ± 0.22
Thr	4.02 ± 0.12	4.00 ± 0.10
Val	4.23 ± 0.10	4.33 ± 0.14
Leu	7.33 ± 0.22	6.51 ± 0.27
Ile	3.06 ± 0.09	2.72 ± 0.14
Phe	3.83 ± 0.12	3.48 ± 0.25
Tyr	2.84 ± 0.10	2.99 ± 0.03
Asp[c]	7.03 ± 0.22	7.03 ± 0.30
Lys	7.74 ± 0.29	6.09 ± 0.02
His	2.55 ± 0.10	1.95 ± 0.04
Arg	6.28 ± 0.16	6.59 ± 0.11
Cys[d]	2.02 ± 0.12	1.74 ± 0.13
Met	1.51 ± 0.06	1.44 ± 0.13
Pro	5.76 ± 0.13	6.99 ± 0.38
OH-Pro	1.66 ± 0.07	3.30 ± 0.20

[a] Values are given as mean ± SEM expressed as grams of amino acid per 16 g nitrogen.
[b] Includes both glutamate and glutamine.
[c] Includes aspartate and asparagine.
[d] Includes both cysteine and cystine.

The rate of fetal nitrogen accretion is important because it is a key factor in determining the nitrogen requirements of the fetus. To this value we must add the rate of fetal nitrogen excretion. We are not certain of all the fetal excretory forms of nitrogen. However, urea excretion via the placenta certainly represents one major form of fetal nitrogen excretion (26). Table 4-3 presents the nitrogen requirement of the fetal lamb estimated from the rate of nitrogen accretion and the rate of urea excretion. Since other forms of nitrogen excretion may exist, this must be regarded as a minimal estimate.

The amino acids of the genetic code have distinctly different metabolic pathways and transport systems. However, they share in common the fact that they serve as building blocks of proteins, that there are no true storage forms of amino acids in the body, and that when not required for protein synthesis, they are oxidized, that is, used as fuels. From a nutri-

Table 4-3

Nitrogen Balance[a]

	Amount (g/kg/day)	Reference
Urea nitrogen excretion	0.36	23
Nitrogen accumulation	0.60	34
Total	0.96	
Umbilical amino acid nitrogen uptake	1.60	32

[a] The fairly large discrepancy between umbilical amino acid nitrogen uptake and nitrogen requirements (1.6 versus 0.96) may represent experimental error and/or not yet measured forms of fetal nitrogen excretion.

tional viewpoint, they are usually subdivided into two groups, essential and nonessential, the division being determined by whether or not there is the potential for their synthesis within the organism. Table 4-1 is subdivided into these two groups. We are not certain whether in early development all nonessential amino acids can be synthesized, or indeed, whether they can be synthesized at rates required to sustain optimal growth. Therefore, it is useful to compare the intake of amino acids by the fetus via the placenta (dietary intake) with the requirements for growth, the latter represented by their accretion rates in protein. The rate of accretion of the essential amino acids represents the absolute minimal rate of placental transport for these amino acids. For the nonessential amino acids, their rates of accretion could be sustained both from the dietary intake of the fetus and from *de novo* synthesis within the fetus. The rate of accretion of individual amino acids is an important reference point in nutrition against which to compare the dietary intake, not only during fetal life, but also during neonatal growth as well. In fetal life the dietary intake is represented by the umbilical uptake, whereas during neonatal life it is represented by the portal venous uptake of nutrients after digestion of the milk provided to the infant.

UPTAKE OF AMINO ACIDS VIA THE UMBILICAL CIRCULATION

The umbilical uptake of amino acids has been measured thus far in only one species, the sheep (35). Table 4-4 presents the mean arteriovenous differences of the individual amino acids across the umbilical $(v - a)$ and uterine $(A - V)$ circulations in the sheep. The necessity for studies of

Table 4-4

Uterine and Umbilical Circulatory Differences of Amino Acids
in the Pregnant Ewe (120 + Days Gestation)[a]

Amino acid	Uterine		Umbilical	
	$A - V$ (mM)	Coefficient extraction (%)	$v - a$ (mM)	Coefficient extraction (%)
Acid				
Asp	1 ± 0.6	3.1	0 ± 0.8	0
Glu	−1 ± 0.9	−1.0	−20 ± 1.2	−14.4
Tau	1 ± 2.3	0.5	0 ± 3.3	0
Neutral				
Gly	4 ± 3.2	0.6	28 ± 10.0	3.4
Ala	12 ± 1.9	6.9	23 ± 4.0	8.7
Thr	8 ± 0.8	7.1	18 ± 4.0	8.7
Ser	10 ± 1.9	8.9	17 ± 3.4	6.3
Val	12 ± 1.5	8.0	26 ± 3.3	7.3
Leu	9 ± 1.9	6.2	22 ± 1.8	10.9
I-Leu	8 ± 1.8	10.1	14 ± 1.6	13.9
Tyr	3 ± 1.1	3.8	13 ± 1.7	6.5
Phe	4 ± 0.8	6.8	12 ± 1.1	10.2
Asn	5 ± 1.7	5.9	14 ± 2.8	18.9
Gln	17 ± 1.5	7.8	49 ± 5.0	13.4
Aba	3 ± 1.2	10.0	1 ± 1.3	4.0
Pro	8 ± 1.4	5.5		
Basic				
Lys	6 ± 1.7	4.6	9 ± 1.4	9.8
His	3 ± 1.0	4.3	3 ± 0.8	6.5
Arg	7 ± 1.4	5.3	20 ± 2.4	21.5
Monomethyl lys	1 ± 1.4	1.5	10 ± 3.3	4.1
3 Me-his	0 ± 0.7	0	4 ± 1.6	5.0
Orn	5 ± 0.6	5.9	4 ± 1.2	4.8
Cit	5 ± 1.1	4.1	5 ± 3.5	3.4
Carn	0 ± 0.9	0	0 ± 4.4	0

[a] Values are given as mean ± SEM.

chronically catheterized unstressed animals is apparent if one compares the arteriovenous differences reported for the same species at the same gestational age from two different laboratories (35, 57); one represents data collected acutely and the other under chronic conditions (Figure 4-1). It is clear that both quantitative and qualitative differences may be introduced by acute stress. This comparison illustrates the difficulty in attempting to interpret amino acid arteriovenous differences across the umbilical circulation in humans since the data are generally collected under

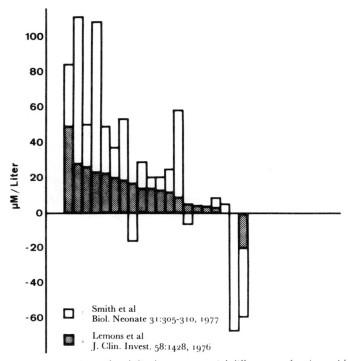

Figure 4-1: A comparison of umbilical venous-arterial differences of amino acids reported in two studies on fetal lambs, one in chronically catheterized animals (35) and one in animals studied acutely (2a, 57). From left to right: glutamine, glycine, valine, alanine, leucine, arginine, threonine, serine, asparagine, isoleucine, tyrosine, phenylalanine, lysine, citrulline, ornithine, 3-methyl histidine, histidine, taurine, asparate, glutamate.

the stress of labor and delivery. It should be emphasized that the differences between data obtained under acute and chronic conditions do not reflect simply a reduction in umbilical and uterine blood flow but also represent changes in metabolism. For if it were only changes in blood flow which distort arteriovenous differences under stress, then the relative magnitude of the arteriovenous difference of each amino acid would be the same in chronic and acute experiments. The fact that some arteriovenous differences are altered more than others implies that there are substantive changes in metabolism as well as changes introduced by alterations in blood flow. For the same reasons, expressing substrate AV differences as metabolic quotients will not correct this problem.

The umbilical venous-arterial differences presented in Table 4-4 were measured in the last 20% of gestation. When they are multiplied by umbilical blood flow, they represent a large uptake of carbon and nitrogen. The total carbon and nitrogen uptake in the form of amino acids is equal to 5.3 g/kg/day of carbon and 1.6 g/kg/day of nitrogen. This represents approximately 60–70% of fetal carbon requirement and approximately 160% of the nitrogen requirement, the latter estimated from nitrogen accretion and urea production. The fact that the nitrogen uptake in the form of amino acids exceeds the nitrogen required for accretion and urea formation suggests that there may be other forms of nitrogen excretion during fetal life. We cannot, however, exclude the possibility that the discrepancy between estimates of nitrogen uptake and requirements is due to experimental error. The extraction coefficients for amino acids across the umbilical and uterine circulations are generally less than 10%, emphasizing the need for both careful quantitative techniques and multiple measurements as discussed in Chapter 3. While it is possible that there is also an umbilical uptake of peptides, it is unlikely that this uptake has nutritional significance since earlier measurements of total α-amino nitrogen uptake are approximately equal in value to the umbilical uptake of amino acids (10).

In the fetal lamb the neutral amino acids are taken up in amounts which exceed their rates of accretion in protein. If one considers only the total quantity of amino acids delivered to the fetus via the umbilical circulation, the glutamine uptake predominates. However, it is important in considering the net uptake of an amino acid by the fetus to compare its uptake with its rate of accretion. Figure 4-2 presents the accretion as a percentage of the umbilical uptake for different amino acids (38). The two basic amino acids, lysine and histidine, and the neutral amino acid, glycine, are delivered to the umbilical circulation in amounts which are barely in excess of their rates of accretion; that is, the rate of accretion equals approximately 70–80% of the umbilical uptake. From a nutritional standpoint, lysine, histidine, and glycine represent amino acids with a potentially narrow margin of safety in the fetus since we are not certain of the rate at which glycine can be synthesized within the fetus and since lysine and histidine are essential amino acids. Presumably a 25–30% reduction in their rates of delivery to the fetus may restrict the net protein accretion rate. The fact that most of the neutral amino acids are provided to the fetus in amounts which far exceed their rates of accretion implies a considerable oxidation rate for these amino acids during fetal life. The issue of the oxidation rate of amino acids and accompanying urea production rate will be discussed later in this chapter. The observation that the neutral amino acids, both essential and nonessential, are provided to the fetus in amounts which far exceed their accretion rates is limited to the fetal lamb and, even in that species, only in late gestation. It would be important to extend the comparison of supply versus accretion rate to other mammals as soon as

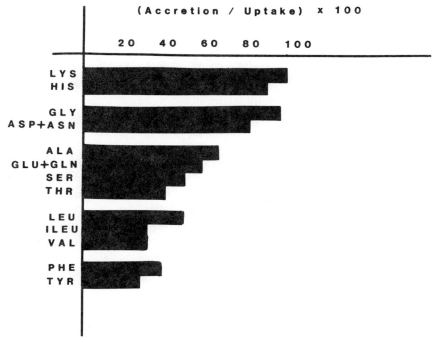

Figure 4-2:   The accretion rate of individual amino acids in the fetal lamb during the latter 20% of gestation expressed as percentage of the umbilical uptake of the amino acid. The accretion rates were obtained from carcass analyses (38), and the umbilical uptakes were measured directly (35). There is an implication of a relatively narrow margin of safety for the basic amino acids.

techniques for measuring umbilical uptake under normal conditions are successfully applied.

The acidic amino acids do not appear to be supplied by the mother to the uterus or by the placenta to the fetus in any appreciable amount. While this has been confirmed by direct measurements only in the ovine fetus (29), studies in subhuman primates have shown very little transport of [¹⁴C]glutamate across the placenta (62). Similarly, in studies with the perfused human placenta, aspartate and glutamate were concentrated on the maternal side (55). Similar data for the relative impermeability of the placenta to glutamate has been obtained in the rat (11). Both aspartate and glutamate are nonessential, and presumably their accretion within fetal proteins is derived from the deamination of glutamine and asparagine. The umbilical uptake of asparagine is more than sufficient to account for the total aspartate and asparagine accretion rate in the fetus. Similarly, the quantity of glutamine entering the umbilical circulation exceeds the total accretion rate of glutamate plus glutamine in the fetus (Figure 4-2). While both asparagine and glutamine are delivered to the fetus in more than adequate amounts to account for their accretion rates, glutamine is not delivered to the uterus from the uterine circulation in amounts equal to the umbilical uptake (29). However, if one adds the glutamate uptake by the placenta from the umbilical circulation and glutamine uptake from the maternal circulation, their combined uptakes are adequate to account for the total quantity of glutamine entering the fetal circulation. Such a calculation implies that glutamate may be transaminated in the placenta, a not unlikely possibility given the high ammonia production rate of the placenta. Figure 4-3 presents the mean umbilical venous-arterial differences for each amino acid versus its corresponding mean uterine arteriovenous difference, the line depicting a relationship of 1.9:1, approximately equal to the proportions of uterine to umbilical blood flows. Within

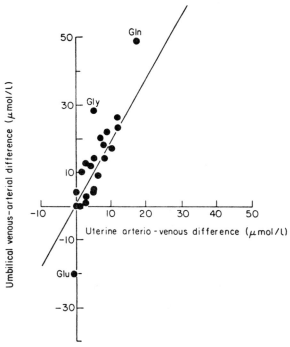

Figure 4-3: Relationship of amino acid venous–arterial differences across the umbilical circulation to arteriovenous differences across the uterine circulation. The regression line includes all points except glycine, glutamine, and glutamate (correlation coefficient = 0.85) (29).

the limits of experimental error, it would appear that most amino acids are taken up by the fetal circulation in amounts approximately equal to their rates of uterine uptake, with little evidence of extensive placental utilization or synthesis at least at this stage in gestation when the placenta is not growing.

FETAL UTILIZATION OF AMINO ACIDS

Fetal Catabolism of Amino Acids

The fact that many amino acids are delivered to the fetal lamb in amounts which exceed their rates of accretion implies a considerable oxidation rate of amino acids in the fetus. This implication receives additional support from the observation that there is a measurable urea concentration difference between fetal and maternal arterial plasma water of approximately 4.5 mg/dl in sheep (26) and approximately 2 mg/dl in humans (25, 51). Since the placental clearance of urea has been measured in sheep (39) and in the subhuman primate (rhesus monkey) (3, 68), the urea production rates by the ovine and human fetus have been estimated as follows:

$$\text{Fetal urea production rate} = (\text{clearance})(a - A)_{\text{urea}}$$

where $(a - A)_{\text{urea}}$ represents the concentration difference of urea between fetal and maternal plasma water. In sheep the clearance can be measured in the same animals in which the $(a - A)_{\text{urea}}$ concentration difference is measured. In humans the urea clearance per kilogram of fetus used in the calculation was that obtained for the rhesus monkey placenta, but this value is not very different from that found in sheep. Table 4-5 presents the

Table 4-5

Urea Production[a]

Placental clearance (ml/kg/min)	Concentration difference: fetal − maternal (mg/100 ml plasma H_2O)	Fetus to placenta diffusion rate (mg/kg/min)
Sheep		
18.8 ± 0.9	4.2 ± 0.4	0.73 ± 0.05
Primates		
15.5 ± 2.1	2.5 ± 0.3[b]	0.39[b] (estimated)

[a] Values are given as mean $\pm$ SEM.
[b] Last two values are for humans.

calculated fetal urea production rate in humans and sheep using this approach. Note that it would be difficult to measure the urea excretion rate from the umbilical circulation by a direct application of the Fick principle because the umbilical extraction coefficient of urea is quite small. However, if [^{14}C]urea is infused into the fetus, a large concentration difference for labeled urea can be created across the placenta, and the umbilical venous–arterial difference of [^{14}C]urea is easily measurable. Under these circumstances, the Fick principle can then be applied to measure the rate of [^{14}C]urea transfer from fetus to mother, and from this the clearance of urea can be calculated (Table 4-6). Thus, although the venous-arterial difference for unlabeled urea is too small to be determined with any precision, the placental transfer of urea produced by the fetus can still be determined indirectly by application of the clearance concept.

In summary, three separate observations have supported the conclusion that there is a considerable oxidation rate of amino acids in the fetal lamb:

1. The umbilical uptake of amino acids exceeds the fetal accretion rate.
2. The uterine uptake of amino acids exceeds the fetal accretion rate.
3. Fetal urea production rate is considerable, exceeding neonatal or adult rates expressed on a per kilogram body weight basis (25, 26, 68).

Table 4-6

**Calculations of Fetal Urea Production
Utilizing Placental Urea Clearance Measurements**[a]

$$\text{Placental urea clearance} = \frac{\text{Umbilical flow} \times (a - v) \, [^{14}\text{C}]\text{urea}}{(a - A) \, [^{14}\text{C}]\text{urea}}$$

$$\text{Fetal urea production} = \text{Placental urea excretion}$$

$$\text{Urea clearance} = \frac{\text{Placental urea excretion}}{(a - A) \, [^{12}\text{C}]\text{urea}}$$

$$\text{Fetal urea production} = \frac{\text{Umbilical flow} \times (a - v) \, [^{14}\text{C}]\text{urea}}{(a - A) \, [^{14}\text{C}]\text{urea}} \times (a - A) \, [^{12}\text{C}]\text{urea}$$

[a] Symbols:

$(a - v) \, [^{14}\text{C}]$urea = arteriovenous concentration difference of [^{14}C]urea in umbilical blood during the constant infusion of [^{14}C]urea into a fetal vein.

$(a - A) \, [^{14}\text{C}]$urea = concentration difference of [^{14}C]urea between fetal arterial and maternal arterial plasma water.

$(a - A) \, [^{12}\text{C}]$urea = concentration difference of urea between fetal arterial and maternal arterial plasma water.

The oxidation rate of an amino acid can be estimated directly with the use of tracer methodology. In fact, tracer methodology provides a powerful analytical tool to define the metabolism of individual amino acids and partition their utilization between oxidation on the one hand and protein synthesis on the other. The key factor for such studies in fetal life is the capability to determine the $^{14}CO_2$ production rate (or $^{13}CO_2$ if stable isotopes of carbon are used) within the fetal compartment. We have tested whether an application of the Fick principle to the umbilical circulation will yield a fairly accurate estimate of $^{14}CO_2$ production (64). $NaH^{14}CO_3$ was infused in fetal lambs at a constant rate, and the infusion rate in dpm/min was compared with the rate leaving the umbilical circulation. The latter was calculated as the product of the umbilical blood flow times the difference in $^{14}CO_2$ concentration between arterial and venous umbilical blood. Approximately 100% (99.6 $\pm$ 1.0%) of the DPMs infused as $NaH^{14}CO_3$ could be recovered as $^{14}CO_2$ leaving the umbilical circulation. Thus, at least in this species, the technology is available to quantify $^{14}CO_2$ production rates within the fetal compartment from the metabolism of ^{14}C-labeled substrates such as amino acids. While this study (64) demonstrated the feasibility of quantifying net $^{14}CO_2$ excretion from the fetal compartment, it also clearly established that the turnover rate of $^{14}CO_2$ calculated as the ratio of the infusion rate of sodium bicarbonate ^{14}C into the fetus to the steady-state fetal arterial CO_2 specific activity was not equivalent to the metabolic production rate of CO_2; in fact, it was five times higher. This discrepancy is important to bear in mind since some investigators have attempted to estimate oxidation rates of nutrients in the fetus not by directly determining the $^{14}CO_2$ excretion rate from the umbilical circulation, but indirectly from the specific activity of $^{14}CO_2$ in fetal plasma.

Since studies on the umbilical uptake of amino acids indicated that the basic amino acids lysine and histidine are delivered to the fetus in amounts which are approximately equal to their net accumulation rates in body proteins (Figure 4-2), it would appear that there is a relatively low rate of catabolism of these essential amino acids in the fetal lamb. To verify this hypothesis, [^{14}C]lysine was infused into the fetus coupled with an infusion of antipyrine for the determination of umbilical blood flow. The $^{14}CO_2$ production rate in the fetal lamb was approximately 9% of the [^{14}C]lysine infusion rate, confirming a relatively low rate of oxidation of this amino acid within the fetus (37). In a subsequent study, partition of leucine fluxes within the fetal lamb was determined using a similar approach of a constant infusion of [^{14}C]leucine into the fetus (65). Figure 4-4 presents in diagrammatic form the results of the leucine studies. Leucine

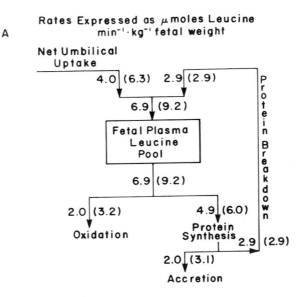

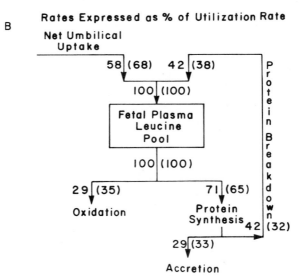

Figure 4-4: Diagram of leucine fluxes into and out of fetal plasma leucine pool. Values in parentheses refer to data collected in mid-gestation fetal lambs (75–90 days gestation); other values refer to data collected in late gestation (120–145 days gestation). A. Weight-specific rates determined in several studies. Note that sum of oxidation and accretion equals net umbilical uptake (31, 65). B. Expresses rates as percentage of utilization. Data from Refs. 31 and 65.

molecules enter the plasma of a 3.2-kg fetus via the placenta and via degradation of fetal proteins with the combined rate of 6.9 μmol/kg/min and exit the fetal plasma to be either oxidized or incorporated into fetal proteins. The oxidation rate is approximately 30% of the total utilization rate (2.0 versus 6.9 μmol/kg/min) and about equal to the net accretion rate in protein. Note that according to this study the high rate of leucine oxidation requires the umbilical uptake of leucine (an essential amino acid) to be approximately twice the accretion rate (4.0 versus 2.0 μmol/kg/min).

More recently fetal leucine fluxes have been studied at mid-gestation when the fetus is approximately 5% of its term weight (31). Even at this early stage of fetal development, there was a high rate of leucine oxidation. Figure 4-4 compares the mean leucine utilization rate, oxidation rate, and protein synthetic rate of the mid-gestation (in parentheses) and late gestation fetuses. The weight-specific leucine oxidation rate is variable in the mid-gestation fetus, but it is at least equal to that of the term fetus. In late gestation the oxidation fraction increases as the leucine concentration in the blood increases, an observation that has been made previously by other investigators for postnatal life.

A number of other studies in fetal physiology have involved the infusion of ^{14}C-labeled amino acids into the fetal circulation and determination of the $^{14}CO_2$ specific activity in fetal blood. As discussed earlier, the experimental design in these studies did not permit a precise determination of the $^{14}CO_2$ production rate since the umbilical $^{14}CO_2$ excretion rate was not directly determined. However, the studies of Hatfield et al. (27) confirmed the appearance of $^{14}CO_2$ in the fetal circulation following the infusion of [^{14}C]alanine and [^{14}C]glycine into the fetal lamb. Similarly, Schaefer and Krishnamurti (53) demonstrated the appearance of $^{14}CO_2$ in the fetal lamb after infusion of [^{14}C]tyrosine. Thus, the oxidation of lysine, leucine, alanine, glycine, and tyrosine by the fetus have all been demonstrated with tracer methodology, and in the case of the first two amino acids, quantitation of the oxidation rate was achieved.

There has been little investigation thus far of what regulates the partition of an amino acid between oxidation and synthesis during fetal life. However, we have found that the oxidation fraction for leucine is increased in the late gestation fetal lamb during a maternal fast (65). This is the first direct evidence of an increased fetal oxidation rate for an amino acid during maternal fasting. This observation is in agreement with those studies which have shown an increased fetal arterial-maternal arterial concentration difference for urea with maternal fasting, an observation which suggested a higher fetal urea production rate under these conditions (34). An important area of study in the years ahead will include the evaluation of those factors, endocrine or trophic, that control the flux of amino acids to protein synthesis or to oxidation.

AMMONIA METABOLISM

The topic of ammonia metabolism is included here since it is an integral part of the description of fetal nitrogen balance. In fact, ammonia metabolism was studied in our laboratory because we hypothesized that NH_3 might represent an additional excretory form of nitrogen for the fetus in addition to urea. Thus, we expected to find a significant efflux of ammonia from the uterus. Figure 4-5 demonstrates that in the pregnant sheep, over most of gestation, this is indeed the case, uterine venous blood having considerably higher ammonia concentration than maternal arterial blood (28). In relation to uterine oxygen uptake, the uterine ammonia excretion is significantly higher in early gestation and decreases toward term. However, to our surprise we found that the ammonia efflux from the uterus does not represent ammonia production within the fetus, but rather production within the uteroplacental tissues. This is demonstrated by the fact that the umbilical venous-arterial differences are positive, thus showing a net uptake of ammonia by the fetus via the umbilical circulation. The situation is analogous to that of lactate in that both ammonia and lactate are small molecules which are produced by the uteroplacental tissues and delivered into both the umbilical and uterine circulations. Just as with lactate production, this appears to be a normal feature of mammalian placental metabolism. *In vitro* both the rat (1, 49) and human placentas (30, 33, 36, 55) have been shown to be sites of ammonia production. Furthermore, in studies in our laboratory ammonia venous-arterial differences have been demonstrated across the uterine circulations in chronically catheterized pregnant rabbits and guinea pigs. Thus, lactate and ammonia production by the uteroplacental tissues have been demonstrated in all mammals studied thus far. As a consequence of the constant infusion of ammonia into the fetal circulation, the arterial blood of the fetus has a relatively high ammonia concentration. It is not clear what the high blood levels of ammonia in the fetus or the constant ammonia infusion from placenta to fetus may mean. However, some clues may be found in studies with isolated adult hepatocytes, which have shown that both lactate and ammonia may be important in directing specific metabolic pathways. Thus, the production rate of ammonia and lactate by the placenta may represent a mechanism by which the placenta influences fetal hepatic metabolism.

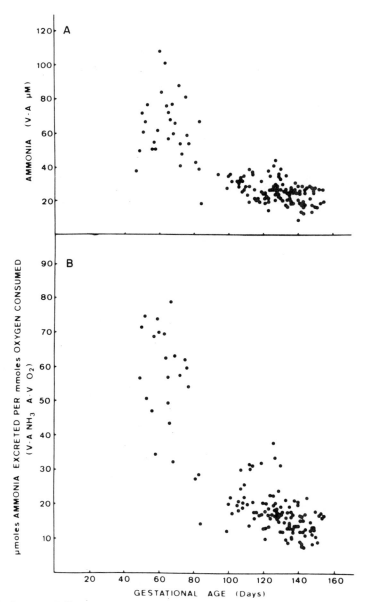

Figure 4-5: A. Difference in ammonia concentration between uterine venous and femoral arterial blood in pregnant sheep from 47 days to term. B. Ammonia (in micromoles) excreted into the maternal circulation per millimole of oxygen consumed by the gravid sheep uterus from 47 days to term (28).

FETAL PROTEIN SYNTHESIS AND TURNOVER

Body proteins are continuously produced and degraded. In a growing animal, the rate of synthesis exceeds the rate of degradation, and there is a net gain of protein mass:

Protein synthetic rate = protein accretion rate + protein degradation

The intravenous infusion of a tracer amino acid can be used to estimate the protein synthetic rate in the whole organism. The simplest procedure, from a conceptual point of view, is to infuse the tracer amino acid at a constant rate until a steady-state specific activity of the free amino acid in blood plasma is attained. At a precisely defined time from the start of the infusion, the animal is killed and the specific activity in body proteins is measured. The fractional synthetic rate (K_s) of body proteins can then be estimated from the steady-state specific activity of the free amino acid (SA_P), the specific activity of the same amino acid in body proteins (SA_{PR}), and the infusion time (t):

$$K_s = SA_{PR}/(SA_P \times t)$$

For example, if the $SA_{PR} : SA_P$ ratio at the end of the infusion is 0.03 and the infusion time is 0.25 day, $K_s = 0.12/\text{day}$, that is, 12% of the body proteins are synthesized each day. This calculation can be made more precise by measuring the rate at which plasma-specific activity attains steady state and by taking into account that, as the tracer amino acid accumulates in the protein pool, there is a recycling of tracer from proteins to plasma due to protein degradation. Whole body protein synthesis measurements can be obtained without killing the animal if the body protein content and amino acid composition are known from previous studies and the transfer rate of the tracer element (e.g., ^{14}C) to other amino acids is negligible. In this case we can assume that at steady state the rate of incorporation of the tracer amino acid into proteins is the difference between the infusion rate and loss of tracer to catabolic pathways. For example, one can infuse [1-^{14}C]leucine and measure the rate of $^{14}CO_2$ excretion, and calculate the rate of [1-^{14}C]leucine incorporation into proteins:

Tracer flux into proteins = tracer infusion − $^{14}CO_2$ excretion

For fetal [1-^{14}C]leucine infusions, however, one must also consider the loss of tracer via the placenta:

Tracer flux into proteins = tracer infusion − $^{14}CO_2$ excretion
− tracer placental loss

The placental loss of tracer amino acid can be quite large (31). In experiments of fetal tracer leucine infusion at mid-gestation, the fraction of tracer leucine infused into the fetus that escaped through the placenta was inversely related to fetal weight, reaching values greater than 60% in the smallest fetuses studied (Figure 4-6). In discussing the results of tracer amino acid studies *in vivo*, it is important to realize the limitations of this type of methodology. Protein synthesis proceeds at quite different rates in different organs and within each organ different proteins have quite different mass and turnover rates. By calculating a protein synthetic rate for the whole organism, we sum individual rates that are markedly different because of individual differences in fractional synthetic rates and in the contribution of any given protein type to total protein mass. Furthermore, protein degradation goes on in every cell of the body so that the specific activity of the traced amino acid at the intracellular sites of utilization can be less than in blood plasma. As a consequence, the protein synthetic rate that is calculated by using plasma specific activity defines only the unidirectional flux of plasma amino acids into protein synthesis. It does not define the total unidirectional flux, because some of the amino acids released by protein degradation within each cell can be utilized without first recycling via the circulating blood. The tendency to underestimate the

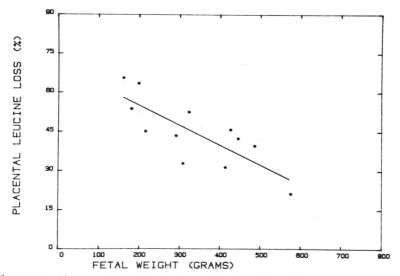

Figure 4-6:   The percentage of the fetal tracer leucine infusion that exits into the uteroplacental and maternal compartments versus fetal weight for mid-gestation (75–90 days) fetal lambs. Note that over 50% of the tracer infusion is lost from the fetal compartment in this manner at mid-gestation. Experimental data from Ref. 31.

total unidirectional flux of an amino acid into protein may be offset to some extent for those amino acids where recycling of tracer may occur. For example, total leucine flux was underestimated by only 10% in adult dogs presumably because of the counteracting errors introduced by recycling of tracer versus entry of unlabeled leucine from protein breakdown (41). Methods that attempt to measure the total flux of amino acids into proteins are outside the scope of our discussion since none of these methods has been applied as yet to fetal studies. In postnatal life, measurements based on plasma-specific activity probably underestimate total protein synthesis by 10–30%. Despite methodologic problems, measurements of protein synthesis in the intact organism have provided important information. In adult mammals protein turnover rate has been shown to be proportional to the three-quarter power of body weight, i.e., to bear the same relationship to body weight as basal energy metabolism (see Table 4-7, protein synthesis (g/kg$^{-0.75}$/day). This means that in small mammals, both the weight-specific oxygen consumption rate and the weight-specific protein turnover rate are higher than in large mammals. In postnatal development the fractional rate of protein synthesis declines as the organism increases in size. Table 4-7 presents data abstracted from the literature by Reeds and Lobley (48a). In part, the inverse relationship between protein turnover and body size is due to the smaller viscera : carcass mass ratio in the larger organism. Viscera such as liver, gut, and kidney have a higher protein turnover rate than skeletal muscle. In postnatal growth, however, there are also major changes in the fractional

Table 4-7

Protein Synthesis (Flux − Amino Acid Catabolism) Estimated with
[I-^{14}C]Leucine in Growing Animals in Energy Balance and in Adults

Species	Body weight (kg)	Protein synthesis (g/day)	Protein synthesis (g/kg/day)	Protein synthesis (g/kg$^{-0.75}$/day)	Reference
Rat growing	0.35	7.7	22.0	16.9	a
Rabbit adult	3.6	39	10.8	14.9	b
Pig growing	30	268	8.9	20.9	c
Sheep adult	63	351	5.6	15.7	d
Human adult	62	279	4.5	12.6	e
Cattle adult	500	1700	3.4	16.1	f

[a] Reeds, P.J., unpublished results.
[b] Lobley, G.E., and Reeds, P.J., unpublished results.
[c] Reeds, P.J., et al., 1980.
[d] Reeds, P.J., Lobley, G.E., and Chalmers, M., unpublished results.
[e] Garlick, P.J., personal communication.
[f] Reeds, P.J., and Orskov, E.R., unpublished results.

protein turnover rates of individual tissues (Table 4-8). Because of these changes and concomitant changes in protein accretion, there are striking developmental variations in protein synthetic rate, as exemplified by Arnal's data on muscle protein synthetic rate in lambs (2). Although growth requires that protein synthesis be in excess of protein degradation, there is no evidence of a decreased rate of protein turnover in growing mammals. The opposite appears to be true since there are several examples of an increased rate of protein degradation during growth. In the same text Waterlow *et al.* (69) pointed out that if one confines the data to those obtained for humans at different stages of development, the protein synthetic rate is higher at early stages of development even when expressed to the three-quarter power of body weight. Thus, within a species, the relationship between body size and protein synthetic rate illustrated in Table 4-7 may not apply.

As discussed earlier, both [^{14}C]lysine and [^{14}C]leucine have been used to study the utilization of these amino acids in the fetal lamb (37, 65). In the studies with radiolabeled lysine, the specific activity of lysine in plasma and in protein hydrolysates prepared from whole body homogenates were determined and a fractional protein synthetic was rate calculated. When similar studies were carried out with [^{14}C]leucine, the two studies provided similar estimates of K_s for the fetal lamb in the latter 20% of gestation. Two key features were confirmed in both studies. First, the fractional protein synthetic rate is much greater than the fractional growth rate (K_G), supporting the observation that there is a high rate of protein turnover in the fetus. Second, K_s is decreasing with increasing gestational age and at a faster rate than K_G. These data are presented in Figure 4-7. In late gestation the rate of protein synthesis was sufficient to account for approximately 25% of the oxygen consumption of the fetus. When the same studies of leucine flux to protein were carried out in the fetal lamb at

Table 4-8

Fractional Synthesis Rate[a,b]

Organ	Young (%/day)	Adult (%/day)	Young ÷ adult (%/day)
Liver	57 ± 12	54 ± 6	95
Kidney	50 ± 10	51 ± 7	102
Brain	17 ± 3	11.3 ± 2.8	66
Heart	18.5 ± 4	11.0 ± 2.3	59
Skeletal muscle	15.2 ± 2.8	4.5 ± 0.5	30

[a] Values given as mean ± SEM.
[b] From Waterlow *et al.* (69).

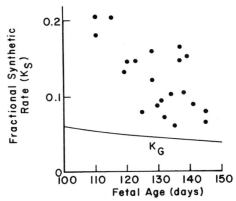

Figure 4-7:   The fractional protein synthetic rate (K_S) is compared to the fractional growth rate (K_G) in fetal lambs from 110 to 145 days gestation. Data from Refs. 37 and 65.

mid-gestation, the leucine utilization rate and protein synthetic rate were greater than in late gestation (expressed as per kilogram of body weight) (31) (Figure 4-4). Since the fetal oxygen consumption per kilogram was also increased in mid-gestation, the higher protein synthetic rate would still only account for approximately 20–25% of the fetal oxygen consumption, just as it does at term.

There have been several other studies carried out in fetal lambs which have attempted to estimate protein synthetic rate for the fetus as a whole (27, 32, 42, 53). However, in all of those studies the disposal rate of an amino acid was not corrected for tracer loss into the placental and maternal compartments nor was a quantitative estimate of the oxidation rate provided. For these reasons it is not surprising that the estimates of protein synthetic rate were two to four times higher than we have outlined.

The decline in fetal protein synthetic rate with advancing gestation is interesting given the fact that there has been considerable debate about the decrease in fetal growth for the human fetus near term. Some investigators have interpreted this slower rate of growth as either artifactual, that is, representing pooling of fetuses growing at different rates, or as representing a limitation of growth rate imposed upon the fetus by the placenta implying a decrease in functional capacity of the placenta relative to the fetal mass. For reasons brought out in discussing the functional maturation of the placenta (Chapter 1), we do not believe that the placenta is imposing a limitation upon fetal growth in a normal pregnancy and prefer to interpret the decrease in protein synthetic rate as one more example of the fetus changing in preparation for parturition.

LIPID METABOLISM

Fat metabolism in fetal life has not been as thoroughly studied as carbohydrate and amino acid metabolism. Most of the studies have centered on the differences in placental permeability to fatty acids and ketoacids with less attention paid to the placental uptake and subsequent hydrolysis of complex lipids.

To review briefly the changes in the maternal concentrations of lipids, there appear to be differences among the species in terms of how maternal lipid concentrations change during pregnancy. However, since not all data were collected under chronic steady-state conditions, these interspecies differences should be interpreted with some caution. In humans it appears that plasma free fatty acid concentrations are slightly increased in the latter part of gestation. In addition, there is evidence that maternal fat depots increase in early gestation and are mobilized and depleted in the latter one-third of gestation, a process which continues through lactation (48). In sheep, guinea pigs, and rabbits studied free of stress there is no significant increase in free fatty acids or ketoacid concentrations during gestation (20, 59). However, the same changes in fat depots may go on, with fat deposition in early pregnancy and mobilization in late pregnancy and during lactation. This has been shown in several different mammalian species (16, 50, 61, 66, 67). Thus, the general pattern is similar across species, namely, a building up of maternal fat depots in early gestation and subsequent mobilization in late gestation.

A general characteristic of pregnancy appears to be the marked increase in blood glycerol, free fatty acids, and ketoacids induced in pregnancy by fasting of even moderate degree. Freinkel and co-workers (17–19) have termed this the *accelerated starvation* induced by pregnancy. There is no question that this phenomenon occurs since it has been well demonstrated in humans, sheep, guinea pigs, rabbits, and rats. Figure 4-8 presents data from the study of Metzger *et al.* in humans, illustrating the striking increases in concentrations of free fatty acids and ketoacids reflecting lipid mobilization and oxidation along with an accompanying maternal hypoglycemia. In the guinea pig these changes can be demonstrated in as little as 2 hr of fasting (21). It is not clear to what extent these changes are brought about by the conceptus acting as a large substrate drain upon the mother, but it seems likely that this is at least partly the explanation. The fact that these changes are so striking in the guinea pig, which has a very large total mass of conceptus, supports this interpretation. Furthermore, if one compares guinea pigs of the same gestational age, two relationships can be clearly established during fasting: (a) the degree of maternal hypoglycemia is directly related to the total fetal mass;

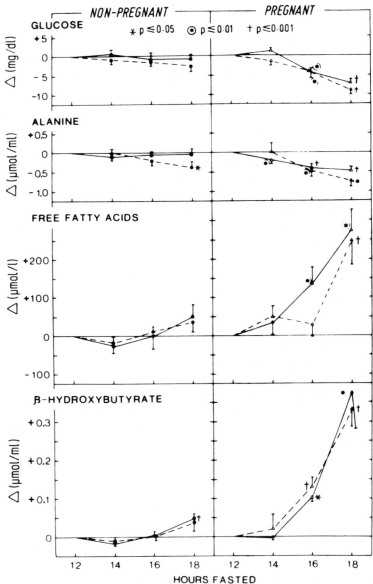

Figure 4-8: Changes in plasma concentrations of glucose, alanine, free fatty acids, and β-hydroxybutyrate in nonpregnant and pregnant women between 12 and 18 hours fast. Values are shown as absolute increments or decrements from the 6:00 AM basal values. (————) Data for obese women; (———) data for lean women. Probabilities given refer to significant differences from 6:00 AM values (40).

and (b) the degree to which maternal glucose utilization is depressed is directly related to the total fetal mass (see Chapter 3). Both of these observations support the hypothesis that placental and fetal metabolic demands account for the phenomenon of accelerated starvation during pregnancy. In sheep the switch to fat mobilization appears to occur around 135 days gestation (67), the quantity of fat mobilized depending upon the litter size and the maternal nutritional level (50).

Once the concentrations of free fatty acids, glycerol and ketoacids are increased in the blood, they are taken up by the uterus and by the fetal circulation to very different degrees depending upon the species. In humans, rabbits, and guinea pigs, the placentas are relatively permeable to these compounds and a correlation can be demonstrated between maternal concentration and fetal uptake. By contrast, the sheep and cat placentas (12) are relatively impermeable to free fatty acids. Figure 4-9 presents such data for humans comparing umbilical venous-arterial differences with the maternal venous concentrations (13).

As we have already pointed out (Chapter 3), there are major technical difficulties in attempting to quantify net free fatty acid uptake by the uterus or by the umbilical circulation under normal physiologic conditions. The precision with which these measurements can be made by any of a variety of techniques does not approach that for glucose, lactate and many other substrates. Furthermore, because of the relatively large molecular weight and high carbon concentration of long chain free fatty acids, a rather small arteriovenous difference across the uterus or placenta (that is, a small coefficient of extraction) may represent a large uptake of substrate. For example, in contrast to lactate for which 1 mmol would require only 3 mmol of oxygen for complete oxidation, 1 mmol of palmitate would require 23 mmol of oxygen. Thus, a coefficient of extraction of 10% in free fatty acid concentrations across the placenta, a coefficient of extraction which may be difficult to measure accurately with current analytical methods, can represent a physiologically significant uptake. A good example of this problem comes from studies in our laboratory describing the metabolic quotients across the guinea pig uterus at approximately 45 days gestation. Table 4-9 demonstrates that the contributions of glucose, lactate, ketoacids, and acetate could not account for more than approximately 80% of the oxygen uptake. Since the guinea pig placenta is readily permeable to free fatty acids, it is likely that they contribute an appreciable part of the missing fraction, but we were unable to demonstrate a statistically significant free fatty acid arteriovenous difference. The mean coefficient of extraction across the uterus was approximately 7%, well within the limits of error of our measurements. Although the coefficient of extraction was small, an arteriovenous difference of

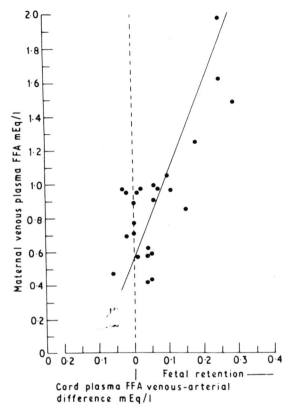

Figure 4-9: Relationship between venous–arterial concentration differences in free fatty acids (FFA) in umbilical cord plasma and maternal concentrations at elective Caesarean section (13).

22 μM (7% coefficient of extraction) for the long chain fatty acids would represent 24% of the uterine oxygen consumption, emphasizing the difficulty in attempting to define net free fatty acid uptake through an application of the Fick principle.

An aspect of lipid metabolism that has not yet been investigated in any systematic way is the contribution to total carbon balance of the uterus made by the uptake of lipids in the form of lipoproteins. Some of the potential pathways for carbon transport to the fetus through free fatty acid or complex lipids include the following: triacylglycerol (TAG) or phospholipids (PPL) could enter the placenta presumably through receptor specific endocytotic mechanisms and either be transferred directly into the fetal circulation or be hydrolyzed within the placenta. There is

Table 4-9

Pregnant Guinea Pig Uterus: Arterial and Venous Concentrations of Oxygen and Substrates and Substrate/Oxygen Quotients[a]

	Oxygen (mM)	Glucose (mM)	Lactate (mM)	Acetoacetate (mM)	BOH butyrate (mM)	Acetate (mM)	Free fatty acids (μM)
Arterial	6.38 ± 0.23	5.26 ± 0.21	1.06 ± 0.09	0.13 ± 0.02	0.13 ± 0.03	0.42 ± 0.04	325 ± 77
Venous	3.84 ± 0.19	4.64 ± 0.21	1.52 ± 0.19	0.12 ± 0.02	0.11 ± 0.02	0.37 ± 0.05	303 ± 74
$A - V$	2.54 ± 0.24	0.62 ± 0.06	0.46 ± 0.12	0.02 ± 0.005	0.02 ± 0.02	0.05 ± 0.01	22 ± 16
	23	13	13	13	13	13	11
Quotient[b]		1.22 ± 0.07	-0.47 ± 0.11	0.01 ± 0.01	0.03 ± 0.02	0.04 ± 0.01	0.24 ± 0.21

[a] Values given as mean $\pm$ SEM.

[b] Glucose + lactate/oxygen quotient = 0.75 (0.13).

also the potential for their hydrolysis at the membrane interface either at the maternal or fetal surfaces. Furthermore, it is possible that complex lipids may be taken up by similar mechanisms from the fetal circulation and undergo similar alternate pathways for metabolism. Figure 4-10 illustrates that net free fatty acid flux across the placenta comes about through three pathways: (a) direct transfer across the placenta, presumably by carrier-specific facilitated diffusion, (b) by *de novo* synthesis within the placenta; and (c) from hydrolysis of TAG or PPL taken up from either the maternal or fetal circulations. Unfortunately, very little is known about these pathways and most of the information which has been collected has been in rats, a species in which chronic steady-state conditions have not yet been established. Thus, at this stage we cannot describe the role that the uptake of complex lipids by the uterus makes to its total carbon balance nor can we quantify the three potential pathways for net free fatty acid transfer to the fetus. It is possible, for example, that complex lipids, once hydrolyzed at the placental surfaces, may be reesterified within the placenta prior to their release into the umbilical circulation.

The synthesis of certain free fatty acids within the placenta has been studied in sheep because the epitheliochorial placenta of the sheep is so impermeable to free fatty acids that it is not clear how the lamb fetus satisfies its requirement of essential fatty acids. This is particularly true with reference to fetal brain growth where there is a relatively large accumulation of the long chain (C-20 to C-22) polyunsaturated ω-6 and ω-3 fatty acids. Crawford *et al.* (9) pointed out that these compounds are not produced to any significant extent in maternal liver. From studies in pregnant guinea pigs in which isotopically labeled linoleic and linolenic acids were administered, they proposed that elongation and desaturation occurred through the interaction of maternal liver, placenta, fetal liver, and fetal brain. In species whose placentas are relatively impermeable to free

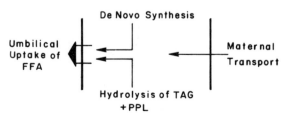

Figure 4-10: Diagram of three potential sources of umbilical free fatty acid (FFA) uptake from the placenta.

fatty acids, this problem of meeting the accretion requirements for normal growth of the fetal brain is accentuated. Noble *et al.* (44) showed the accumulation of the n-9 eicosatrienoic acid, a marker of essential fatty acid deficiency, within the fetal lamb circulation. In earlier studies Noble *et al.* had shown the rapid decrease in the ratio of eicosatrienoic acid/ arachidonic acid in the tissues of the lamb from fetal life to the tenth day of postnatal life (43). These same investigators have provided convincing evidence that the sheep placenta can desaturate and chain elongate free fatty acids (44). They demonstrated high $\Delta 9$- and $\Delta 6$-desaturase activity within the sheep placenta and appreciable conversion of the 1-^{14}C $18:0$ substrate to a $20:4$ substrate and intermediate desaturated fatty acids (56). Thus, the sheep placenta, while relatively impermeable to free fatty acids, may be quite active metabolically in the synthesis of the longer chain desaturated fatty acids. Zimmerman *et al.* (71) have provided some evidence of *de novo* synthesis of arachidonic acid from [^{14}C]acetate in both human and rat placentas.

A comparison among species of fetal fat accretion with placental permeability to free fatty acids has brought out the interesting point that species such as humans and guinea pigs, which produce newborns with high concentrations of body fat, have placentas relatively permeable to free fatty acids. Whether the main fate of free fatty acids in these species is accretion, both in structural phospholipids and in storage of triacylglycerol, or whether they contribute significantly as fuels of energy metabolism is not yet clear.

After birth, milk provides a relatively high fat diet compared to that consumed by the fetus, and it is clear that lipids play an important role both as fuels and in fat deposition. On this latter point Clandinin *et al.* (6– 8) have begun to use the approach described in the section on amino acid metabolism, namely, that of taking as a reference point the accretion rate of essential fatty acids during normal growth of the human fetus and newborn and comparing dietary intake against the background of this accretion rate. Their data demonstrate a lag in accretion of long chain polyenic essential fatty acids in both the brain and liver during fetal development, with mobilization of essential fatty acid depots in the liver for a varying period after delivery. From such data, they estimate that a premature infant of approximately 1300 g might have essential fatty acid reserves in the liver to meet normal growth and accretion rates of the brain for 2–9 days depending upon the fatty acid group selected. Certainly further work needs to be done in a variety of species including humans to define the capacity of the liver and placenta for synthesis of the long chain polyenic fatty acids.

POSTNATAL FAT METABOLISM

For most mammalian species birth represents an abrupt transition from a low to a high fat diet. Even in those species with placentas relatively permeable to free fatty acids, milk produced by the mammary gland represents a rich fat diet. Figure 4-11 compares the milk of a few species with that of the umbilical uptake of nutrients in the fetal lamb during late gestation. The species whose breast milk is compared to the "fetal milk" include sheep and humans as well as several aquatic mammals. The latter are included to illustrate that in those mammals where water conservation is important to the mother (e.g., aquatic and desert mammals), the milk contains a very high concentration of fat. However, even in sheep and in humans, milk represents a high fat diet particularly when contrasted with the nutrients provided *in utero* to the fetal lamb. Thus, the transition from fetal to neonatal life represents a move to a relatively high fat diet. Furthermore, not only is the provision of fat different, but the utilization of fatty acids is different, with little evidence that free fatty acids are oxidized during fetal life, whereas there is an extensive oxidation of fatty acids during neonatal life.

The endocrine changes which occur at birth, particularly the surge in glucagon concentration leading to a much lower insulin : glucagon ratio than in fetal life, favor the mobilization of lipids from peripheral tissues and, as free fatty acids and glycerol concentrations in the blood increase, a higher rate of free fatty acid oxidation in the liver leading to an increasing ketone body concentration. These changes in neonatal life have been well described in a number of species including humans, rats, rabbits, and

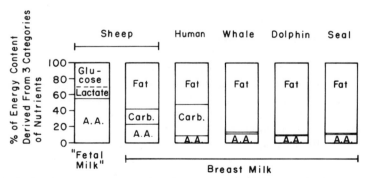

Figure 4-11: Diagram comparing the relative energy contributions of carbohydrates, fats, and amino acids to the milk produced in humans, sheep, and several aquatic mammals. "Fetal milk" refers to the umbilical uptake of the major carbon and nitrogen sources in the late gestation fetal lamb.

pigs (22, 24, 47). In all species there is an appreciable lag before the concentrations of β-hydroxybutyrate and acetoacetate rise following the increase in free fatty acid concentrations. In humans the infant is born with large white fat depots, and therefore, it is not surprising that these changes are easily demonstrated (46). The importance of these changes in newborn metabolic homeostasis has been clarified in recent years, particularly in terms of the importance of the oxidation of fatty acids for the maintenance of a normal blood glucose concentration.

When the newborn begins milk feedings, there is not only an increase in fat intake but a sudden alteration in glucose intake. During fetal life glucose is supplied continuously from the placenta and in relatively large amounts. The principal sugar in milk is lactose. In human milk its concentration is approximately 7%. Thus, an infant consuming 150 ml/kg/day of milk has a glucose intake of only 5.5 g/kg/day. Therefore, the infant must increase its glucose production rate sharply. The oxidation of fatty acids in the liver is essential to maintain a high gluconeogenic rate. This has been demonstrated in a number of ways.

When newborn rabbits are fasted, a profound hypoglycemia develops. The hypoglycemia is not corrected by the provision of carbon precursors for glucose such as lactate or gluconeogenic amino acids. However, if both the gluconeogenic precursors and fat are provided, the glucose concentration is restored to the normal level (45). This is not due primarily to an effect of fat sparing the peripheral utilization of glucose since the glucose disappearance rate following a bolus injection is not altered by the fat administration. Rather, this effect of fat supply upon glucose concentrations reflects the fact that the oxidation of fats in the liver sustains the high rate of gluconeogenesis (14, 15). If long chain fatty acid oxidation is blocked with inhibitors such as tetradecylglycidic acid (TDGA) (23) or McN-3716 (63), the hypoglycemia is not corrected. However, a rapid correction of hypoglycemia occurs when the block of fatty acid oxidation is circumvented by medium chain triglycerides (63). Their rapid oxidation is associated with the appearance of their oxidation products, β-hydroxybutyrate and acetoacetate as well as an increase in the blood glucose concentration (Figures 4-12A and B). Thus, whenever there is a restriction in the rate of oxidation of long chain fatty acids in the neonatal period, as for example, from a relative carnitine deficiency or acyl carnitine transferase deficiency, a hypoglycemia develops in spite of an adequate supply of glucose precursors to the liver. This hypoglycemia can be prevented or corrected by the introduction of medium chain triglycerides which circumvent this block by entering the mitochondria directly and restoring fatty acid oxidation, which in turn fuels a high rate of gluconeogenesis and restores the blood sugar concentration. These processes are

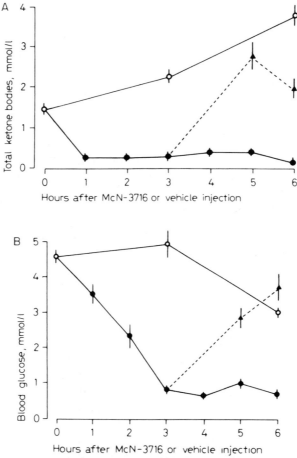

Figure 4-12:   A. Blood ketone bodies (acetoacetate + β-hydroxybutyrate) in suckling rats after McN-3716 injection and medium chain triglycerides (MCT) feeding. Sucking rats were injected with McN-3716 (●) or with the vehicle alone (O), or were injected with McN-3716 and fed 3 hr later with MCT (▲). Results are the means ± SEM of 8–10 determinations. B. Blood glucose in suckling rats after McN-3716 injection and MCT feeding. Suckling rats were injected with McN-3716 (●) or with the vehicle alone (O) or were injected with McN-3716 and fed 3 hr later with MCT (▲). Results are the means ± SEM of 8–10 determinations (63).

as important in newborn infants as they are in neonatal animals. Sann *et al.* (52) have shown similar relationships between fat intake and glucose concentration and clearance in preterm infants. Similarly, Bougneres *et al.* (5) observed that a child with a block in long chain fatty acid oxidation became hypoglycemic with fasting. By the administration of medium chain triglycerides the hypoglycemia was rapidly corrected and ketone body concentration increased concomitantly. Schmidt-Sommerfeld *et al.* (54) have provided supporting evidence of a potential carnitine deficiency in newborn infants by the change in free fatty acid : ketone body ratio induced by dietary supplementation with carnitine. These seem to be more than adequate reasons to include medium chain triglycerides as part of the dietary fat intake in both preterm and full term infants.

The transition from a fetal diet derived from the placenta to a milk diet and the subsequent transition during postnatal life from a milk diet to the diet characteristic of that species in adult life needs further study, particularly in the relationship between fat intake, lipogenesis, and fat mobilization. The factors responsible during fetal life for diverting free fatty acids away from oxidation and toward fat accretion have also not yet been identified.

REFERENCES

1. Adachi, H. (1967). *The placenta and hormones.* Journal of Japanese Obstetrics and Gynecologic Society **19,** 665–669.
2. Arnal, M. (1977). *Muscle protein turnover in lambs throughout development. In* "Protein Metabolism and Nutrition: Proceedings of the International Symposium on Protein Metabolism and Nutrition," 2nd edition, pp 38–40, Flevohof, Holland.
2a. Battaglia, F.C. (1979). *Umbilical uptake of substrates and their role in fetal metabolism. In* "Nutrition and Metabolism of the Fetus and Infant," Fifth Nutricia Symposium, (H.K.A. Visser, ed.), pp. 83–91, Martinus Nijhoff Publishers, The Hague, the Netherlands.
3. Battaglia, F.C., Behrman, R.E., Meschia, G., Seeds, A.E. and Bruns, P.D. (1968). *Clearance of inert molecules, Na, and Cl ions across the primate placenta.* American Journal of Obstetrics and Gynecology, **102,** 1135–1143.
4. Blaxter, K.L. (1962). "The Energy Metabolism of Ruminants." C. Thomas Publishers, Springfield, Illinois.
5. Bougneres, P.-F., Saudubray, M.-M., Marsac, C., Bernard, O., Odievre, M. and Girard, J. (1981). *Fasting hypoglycemia resulting from hepatic carnitine palmitoyl transferase deficiency.* Journal of Pediatrics **98,** 742–746.
6. Clandinin, M.T., Chappell, J.E., Leong, S., Heim, T., Swyer, P.R. and Chance, G.W. (1980). *Intrauterine fatty acid accretion rates in human brain: implications for fatty acid requirements.* Early Human Development **4/2,** 121–129.
7. Clandinin, M.T., Chappell, J.E., Leong, S., Heim, T., Swyer, P.R. and Chance, G.W. (1980). *Extrauterine fatty acid accretion in infant brain: implications for fatty acid requirements.* Early Human Development **4/2,** 131–138.
8. Clandinin, M.T., Chappell, J.E., Heim, T., Swyer, P.R. and Chance, G.W. (1981). *Fatty acid accretion in fetal and neonatal liver: implications for fatty acid requirements.* Early Human Development **5,** 7–14.
9. Crawford, M.A., Hassam, A.G., Williams, G. and Whitehouse, W.L. (1976). *Essential fatty acid and fetal brain growth.* Lancet **1,** 452–453.

10. deBella, G. (1958). *A comparative study of the concentrations of nonprotein, urea, and amino acid nitrogen in the maternal and fetal plasmas of sheep and goats.* Yale Journal of Biology and Medicine **30**, 368–373.
11. Dierks-Ventling, C., Cone, A.L. and Wapnir, R.A. (1971). *Placental transfer of amino acids in the rat. I. l-glutamic acid and l-glutamine.* Biology of the Neonate **17**, 361–372.
12. Elphick, M.C. and Hull, D. (1984). *Transfer of fatty acid across the cat placenta.* Journal of Developmental Physiology **6**, 517–525.
13. Elphick, M.C., Hull, D. and Sanders, R.R. (1976). *Concentrations of free fatty acids in maternal and umbilical cord blood during elective Caesarean section.* British Journal of Obstetrics and Gynaecology **83**, 539–544.
14. Ferre, P., Satabin, P., El Manoubi, L., Callikan, S. and Girard, J. (1981). *Relationship between ketogenesis and gluconeogenesis in isolated hepatocytes from newborn rats.* Biochemical Journal **200**, 429–433.
15. Ferre, P., Satabin, P., Decaux, J.-F., Escriva, F. and Girard, J. (1983). *Development and regulation of ketogenesis in hepatocytes isolated from newborn rats.* Biochemical Journal **214**, 937–942.
16. Flint, D.J., Sinnett-Smith, P.A., Clegg, R.A. and Vernon, R.G. (1979). *Role of insulin receptors in the changing metabolism of adipose tissue during pregnancy and lactation in the rat.* Biochemistry Journal **182**, 421–427.
17. Freinkel, N. and Metzger, B.E. (1975). *Some considerations of fuel economy in the fed state during late human pregnancy.* In "Early Diabetes in Early Life," (R.A. Camerini-Davalos and H.S. Cole, eds.), pp 289–301, Academic Press, New York.
18. Freinkel, N. and Metzger, B.E. (1979). *Pregnancy as a tissue culture experience: the critical implications of maternal metabolism for fetal development. In* "Pregnancy Metabolism, Diabetes and the Fetus," Ciba Foundation Symposium 63, pp 3–23, Excerpta Medica, Amsterdam.
19. Freinkel, N., Phelps, R.L. and Metzger, B.E. (1979). *Intermediary metabolism during normal pregnancy. In* "Carbohydrate Metabolism in Pregnancy and the Newborn," (H.W. Sutherland and J.M. Stowers, eds.), 2nd Aberdeen Int. Colloq., Springer, Berlin.
20. Gilbert, M., Hay, W.W. Jr., Johnson, R.L. and Battaglia, F.C. (1984). *Some aspects of maternal metabolism throughout pregnancy in the conscious rabbit.* Pediatric Research **18**, 854–859.
21. Gilbert, M., Sparks, J.W. and Battaglia, F.C. (1985). *Effects of fasting on glucose turnover rate and metabolite levels in conscious pregnant guinea pigs.* Biology of the Neonate **48**, 85–89.
22. Girard, J. (1981). *Fuel homeostasis during the perinatal period. In* "The Biology of Normal Human Growth" (M. Ritzen, et al, eds.), pp 193–202, Raven Press, New York.
23. Girard, J. (1982). *Gluconeogenesis and the regulation of blood glucose concentration in the newborn. In* "Diabetes 1982," Proceedings of the 11th Congress of the International Diabetes Foundation, International Congress Series No. 600 (E.N. Mangola, ed.), pp 417–421, Excerpta Medica, Amsterdam.
24. Girard, J.R., Ferre, P., Kervran, A., Pegorier, J.P. and Assan, R. (1977). *Role of insulin/glucagon ratio in the changes of hepatic metabolism during development of the rat. In* "Glucagon: Its Role in Physiology and Clinical Medicine" (P.P. Foa, J.S. Bajaj and N.L. Foa, eds.), pp 563–581, Springer-Verlag, New York.
25. Gresham, E.L., Simons, P.S. and Battaglia, F.C. (1971). *Maternal-fetal urea concentration difference in man: Metabolic significance.* Journal of Pediatrics **79**, 809–811.
26. Gresham, E.L., James, E.J., Raye, J.R., Battaglia, F.C., Makowski, E.L. and Meschia, G. (1972). *Production and excretion of urea by the fetal lamb.* Pediatrics **50**, 372–379.
27. Hatfield, G.M., Joyce, J., Jeacock, M.K. and Shepherd, D.A.L. (1984). *The irreversible*

loss of alanine and of glycine in fetal and sucking lambs. British Journal of Nutrition **52**, 529–543.

28. Holzman, I.R., Lemons, J.A., Meschia, G. and Battaglia, F.C. (1977). *Ammonia production by the pregnant uterus*. Proceedings of the Society for Experimental Biology and Medicine **156**, 27–30.

29. Holzman, I.R., Lemons, J.A., Meschia, G. and Battaglia, F.C. (1979). *Uterine uptake of amino acids and glutamine-glutamate balance across the placenta of the pregnant ewe*. Journal of Developmental Physiology **1**, 137–149.

30. Holzman, I.R., Philipps, A.F. and Battaglia, F.C. (1979). *Glucose metabolism and ammonia production by the human placenta in vitro*. Pediatric Research **13**, 117–120.

31. Kennaugh, J.M., Bell, A.W., Battaglia, F.C. and Meschia, G. (In preparation). *Ontogenetic changes in leucine disposal rate, oxidation rate, and protein synthetic rate during fetal life.*

32. Kitts, D.D. and Krishnamurti, C.R. (1982). *Kinetics of amino acid metabolism in the ovine fetus in utero*. Growth **46**, 209–219.

33. Kodama, I. (1972). *Studies on ammonia metabolism of placenta*. Journal of Japanese Obstetrics and Gynecologic Society **24**, 155–164.

34. Lemons, J.A. and Schreiner, R.L. (1984). *Metabolic balance of the ovine fetus during the fed and fasted states*. Annals of Nutrition and Metabolism **28**, 268–280.

35. Lemons, J.A., Adcock, E.W. III, Jones, M.D. Jr., Naughton, M.A., Meschia, G. and Battaglia, F.C. (1976). *Umbilical uptake of amino acids in the unstressed fetal lamb*. Journal of Clinical Investigation **58**, 1428–1434.

36. Luschinsky, H.L. (1951). *The activity of glutaminase in the human placenta*. Archives of Biochemistry and Biophysics **31**, 132–140.

37. Meier, P.R., Peterson, R.B., Bonds, D.R., Meschia, G. and Battaglia, F.C. (1981). *Rates of protein synthesis and turnover in fetal life*. American Journal of Physiology **240**, E320–E324.

38. Meier, P.R., Teng, C., Battaglia, F.C. and Meschia, G. (1981). *The rate of amino acid nitrogen and total nitrogen accumulation in the fetal lamb*. Proceedings of the Society for Experimental Biology and Medicine **167**, 463–468.

39. Meschia, G., Battaglia, F.C. and Bruns, P.D. (1967). *Theoretical and experimental study of transplacental diffusion*. Journal of Applied Physiology **22**, 1171–1178.

40. Metzger, B.E., Vileisis, R.A., Ravnikar, V. and Freinkel, N. (1982). *"Accelerated starvation" and the skipped breakfast in late normal pregnancy*. The Lancet **1**, 588–592.

41. Nissen, S. and Haymond, M.W. (1981). *Effects of fasting on flux and interconversion of leucine and alpha-ketoisocaproate in vivo*. American Journal of Physiology **241**, E72–E75.

42. Noakes, D.E. and Young, M. (1981). *Measurement of fetal tissue protein synthetic rate in the lamb in utero*. Research in Veterinary Science **31**, 336–341.

43. Noble, R.C., Steele, W. and Moore, J.H. (1972). *The metabolism of linoleic acid by the young lamb*. British Journal of Nutrition **27**, 503–508.

44. Noble, R.C., Shand, J.H. and Christie, W.W. (1985). *Synthesis of C20 and C22 polyunsaturated fatty acids by the placenta of the sheep*. Biology of the Neonate **47**, 333–338.

45. Pegorier, J.P., Leturque, A., Ferre, P., Turlan, P. and Girard, J. (1983). *Effects of medium-chain triglyceride feeding on glucose homeostasis in the newborn rat*. American Journal of Physiology **244**, E329–E334.

46. Persson, B. and Gentz, J. (1966). *The pattern of blood lipids, glycerol and ketone bodies during the neonatal period, infancy and childhood*. Acta Paediatrica Scandinavia **55**, 465–473.

47. Persson, B., Feychting, H. and Gentz, S. (1975). *Management of the infant of the diabetic mother. In* "Carbohydrate Metabolism in Pregnancy and the Newborn," (W.H. Sutherland and J.M. Stowers, eds.), pp 232–248, Churchill Livingstone, Edinburgh.

48. Pipe, N.G.J., Smith, T., Halliday, D., Edmonds, C.J., Williams, C. and Coltart, T.M. (1979). *Changes in fat, fat-free mass and body water in human normal pregnancy.* British Journal of Obstetrics and Gynaecology **86**, 929–940.

48a. Reeds, P.J. and Lobley, G.E. (1980). *Protein synthesis: are there real species differences?* Proceedings of the Nutrition Society **39**, 43–52.

49. Remesar, X., Arola, L., Palou, A. and Alemany, M. (1980). *Activities of enzymes involved in amino-acid metabolism in developing rat placenta.* European Journal of Biochemistry **110**, 289–293.

50. Robinson, J.J., MacDonald, I., McHatti, I. and Pennie, K. (1978). *Studies on reproduction in prolific ewes. 4. Sequential changes in maternal body during pregnancy.* Journal of Agricultural Science **91**, 291–304.

51. Rubaltelli, F.F. and Formentin, P.A. (1968). *Ammonia nitrogen, urea, and uric acid blood levels in the mother and in both umbilical vessels at delivery.* Biology of the Neonate **13**, 147–154.

52. Sann, L., Mathieu, M., Lasne, Y. and Ruitton, A. (1981). *Effect of oral administration of lipids with 67% medium chain triglycerides on glucose homeostasis in preterm neonates.* Metabolism **30**, 712–716.

53. Schaefer, A.L. and Krishnamurti, C.R. (1984). *Whole body and tissue fractional protein synthesis in the ovine fetus in utero.* British Journal of Nutrition **52**, 359–369.

54. Schmidt-Sommerfeld, E., Penn, D. and Wolf, H. (1983). *Carnitine deficiency in premature infants receiving total parenteral nutrition: Effect of L-carnitine supplementation.* Journal of Pediatrics **102**, 931–935.

55. Schneider, H., Mohlen, K.-H. and Dancis, J. (1979). *Transfer of amino acids across* in vitro *perfused human placenta.* Pediatric Research **13**, 236–240.

56. Shand, J.H. and Noble, R.C. (1979). *$\Delta 9$- and $\Delta 6$-desaturase activities of the ovine placenta and their role in the supply of fatty acids to the fetus.* Biology of the Neonate **36**, 298–304.

57. Smith, R.M., Jarrett, I.G., King, R.A. and Russell, G.R. (1977). *Amino acid nutrition of the fetal lamb.* Biology of the Neonate **31**, 305–310.

58. Southgate, D.A.T. (1971). *The accumulation of amino acids in the products of conception of the rat and in the young animal after birth.* Biology of the Neonate **19**, 272–292.

59. Sparks, J.W., Pegorier, J.-P., Girard, J. and Battaglia, F.C. (1981). *Substrate concentration changes during pregnancy in the guinea pig studied under unstressed steady state conditions.* Pediatric Research **15**, 1340–1344.

60. Sparks, J.W., Girard, J.R., Callikan, S. and Battaglia, F.C. (1985). *Growth of the fetal guinea pig: Physical and chemical characteristics.* American Journal of Physiology **248**, E132–E139.

61. Spray, R.W. (1973). British Journal of Nutrition **4**, 354–360.

62. Steigink, L.D., Pitkin, R.M., Reynolds, W.A., Filer, L.J. Jr., Boaz, D.P. and Brummel, M.C. (1975). *Placental transfer of glutamate and its metabolites in the primate.* American Journal of Obstetrics and Gynecology **122**, 70–78.

63. Turlan, P., Ferre, P. and Girard, J.R. (1983). *Evidence that medium-chain fatty acid oxidation can support an active gluconeogenesis in the suckling newborn rat.* Biology of the Neonate **43**, 103–108.

64. van Veen, L.C.P., Hay, W.W. Jr., Battaglia, F.C. and Meschia, G. (1984). *Fetal CO_2 kinetics.* Journal of Developmental Physiology **6**, 359–365.

65. van Veen, L.C.P., Meschia, G., Hay, W.W. Jr. and Battaglia, F.C. (In preparation). *Leucine disposal and oxidation rates in the fetal lamb.*

66. Vernon, R.G. (1980). *Lipid metabolism in the adipose tissue of ruminant animals.* Progress in Lipid Research **19,** 23–106.

67. Vernon, R.G., Clegg, R.A. and Flint, D.J. (1981). *Metabolism of sheep adipose tissue during pregnancy and lactation. Adaptation and regulation.* Biochemistry Journal **200,** 307–314.

68. Wallenburg, H.C. and van Kreel, B.K. (1977). *Placental and nonplacental drainage of the uterus in the pregnant rhesus monkey.* European Journal of Obstetrics, Gynecology and Reproductive Biology **7,** 79–84.

69. Waterlow, J.C., Garlick, P.J. and Millward, D.J. (1978). "Protein Turnover in Mammalian Tissues and in the Whole Body." Elsevier/North-Holland Biomedical Press, Amsterdam.

70. Williams, H.H., Curtin, L.V., Abraham, J., Loosli, J.B. and Maynard, L.A. (1954). *Estimation of growth requirements for amino acids by assay of the carcass.* Journal of Biologic Chemistry **208,** 277–286.

71. Zimmerman, T., Winkler, L., Moller, U., Schubert, H. and Goetze, E. (1979). *Synthesis of arachidonic acid in the human placenta in vitro.* Biology of the Neonate **35,** 209–212.

5

Individual Organ Metabolism
in the Fetus

The metabolism of individual organs has only recently begun to be explored in a systematic way in fetal physiology. It is impressive, however, that as many as six different fetal organs or tissue beds have been studied in a single species, the sheep, and some of their metabolic quotients delineated under chronic steady-state conditions. This constitutes more information about individual organs than has been collected for the newborn; since these different organs have been studied in the same species, we are beginning to be able to construct a fairly comprehensive picture of fetal metabolism.

Several important questions in perinatal biology are addressed by such studies. First, it is important to define under physiologic conditions how the metabolism of an organ changes during development. Second, metabolism and organ function are intertwined, so that the metabolic changes induced by development have functional implications as well. Third, as a fairly complete description of the metabolism of the major organs is obtained, one can begin to construct the metabolism of the whole organism from its individual parts and compare this construction with data obtained by direct metabolic studies of the whole animal. For example, in previous chapters of this book we described the methodology which permits determination of fetal glucose utilization and production rates. One should arrive at similar estimates by adding the utilization and/or production rates of glucose for each of the major organs of the fetal body. Such internal consistency in metabolic data has been difficult to achieve even for adult animals. If it were attained for the fetus, however, it would certainly strengthen our confidence in the estimates of metabolic fluxes made for the whole fetal organism and each of its individual organs.

CARCASS METABOLISM

It seems appropriate to begin with the data on carcass (i.e., nonvisceral) metabolism since the carcass represents a large proportion of the tissues of the body. In postnatal life the fraction of the body weight represented by skin, muscle, and skeleton varies with body size. In the larger animals the carcass is a greater percentage of body weight since it must play a larger role in supporting the body. The relationship between visceral organs versus carcass has not been well described for fetal life, but presumably the proportion which is carcass could be considerably less in the immature fetus given the absence of any requirement for support against gravity. In the mature fetal lamb, however, carcass already represents approximately 70% of body weight.

Studies have been carried out in which metabolic quotients were obtained simultaneously for the hind limb of the pregnant ewe and the hind limb of her fetus (30, 31). The studies demonstrate that the hind limb has a much higher glucose/oxygen quotient in the fetus than in the adult sheep, despite the much lower arterial glucose concentration of fetal blood (Figure 5-1). Furthermore, in both mother and fetus hind limb, glucose arteriovenous differences decrease as the blood glucose decreases below normal levels during a maternal fast (Figure 5-2).

Figure 5-3 taken from the same study demonstrates that at comparable levels of arterial oxygen content the fetal hind limb has a much smaller arteriovenous difference of oxygen. In fact, fetal hind limb has an oxygen arteriovenous difference approximately one-third that of the adult hind limb. Since the reciprocal of the arteriovenous difference in oxygen content is a measure of the quantity of blood which must perfuse the tissue per millimole of oxygen consumed, Figure 5-3 implies that the fetal carcass is perfused at a rate which is approximately three times that of adult tissues with respect to its oxygen requirements. This is true of other fetal organs as well. The higher rate of perfusion of fetal tissues is one of the major mechanisms by which the fetal lamb can maintain a relatively high rate of glucose and oxygen utilization despite very low glucose concentrations and oxygen tensions in fetal arterial blood.

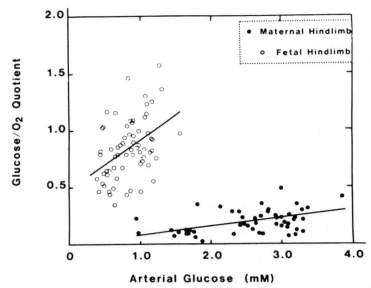

Figure 5-1: Relationship of arterial glucose concentration to glucose/oxygen quotient in fetal (O) and maternal (●) hind limbs. Maternal hind limb: $y = 0.074x + 0.01$, $n = 55$, $p = 0.45$; fetal hind limb: $y = 0.43x + 0.48$, $n = 67$, $p < 0.45$ (30, 31).

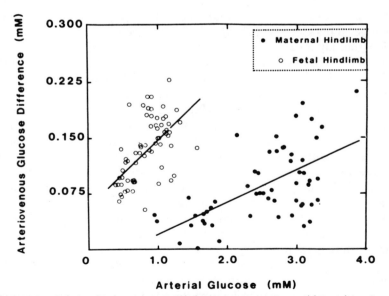

Figure 5-2: Relationship between arterial glucose concentration and femoral arteriovenous difference in fetal (O) and maternal (●) hind limbs. Maternal hind limb: $y = 0.04x - 0.02$, $p < 0.59$, $n = 55$; fetal hind limb: $y = 0.09x + 0.06$, $n = 67$, $p < 0.57$ (30, 31).

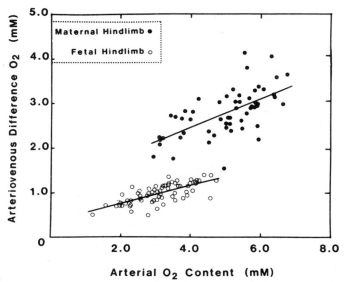

Figure 5-3: Relationship between arterial oxygen content and arteriovenous differences of oxygen across both fetal (O) and maternal (●) hind limbs. Maternal hind limb: $y = 0.32x + 1.18$, $p < 0.63$, $n = 56$; fetal hind limb: $y = 0.20x + 0.36$, $n = 67$, $p < 0.71$ (30, 31).

Jarrett *et al.* (16) studied metabolic quotients across the hind limb of adult sheep. Their data presented in Figure 5-4 demonstrate that the glucose/oxygen quotient decreases with fasting and increases with exercise. Figure 5-5 compares metabolic quotients for several substrates across the fetal and maternal limbs while the mother was standing quietly in a stall (30, 31). The glucose + lactate/oxygen quotient across the maternal hind limb in the study was only 0.12, which compares favorably with the 0.08 quotient found by Jarrett *et al.* in resting, nonpregnant ewes. By contrast, the fetal hind limb glucose + lactate/oxygen quotient was 0.68, indicating that the high glucose uptake by the fetal limbs is not simply due to high lactate production. Nevertheless, there is a significant lactate output from the fetal hind limb (lactate/oxygen quotient = -0.14 ± 0.03). Liechty and Lemons (22) also reported relatively high glucose/oxygen quotients across the hind limb of the fetal lamb. They found the mean glucose/oxygen quotient to be 1.20 in the fed state and significantly less (0.621) on the fifth day of fasting. No lactate/oxygen quotients across the limb were determined in this study, so a net glucose + lactate/oxygen quotient could not be calculated. In earlier chapters we pointed out the following two characteristics of normal fetal lactate metabolism: (a) the fetus as a whole is a net consumer of lactic acid since there is a net fetal uptake of lactic acid via the umbilical circulation, and (b) lactate is produced within the

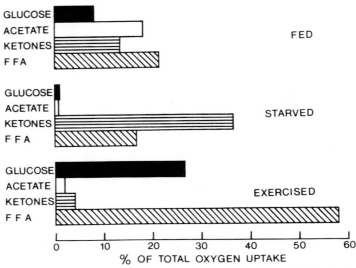

Figure 5-4: The percentage of the oxygen uptake by the sheep hind limb that can be accounted for if the various metabolic fuels are completely oxidized to CO_2 and H_2O. Molar glucose uptake has been reduced by half the molar lactate output. In these calculations it has been assumed that complete oxidation of each mole of nutrient requires the following number of moles of oxygen: acetate, 2; glucose, 6; acetoacetate, 4; β-hydroxybutyrate, 4.5; free fatty acids, 23. Values for the exercising animals are for the sheep walking on a 15° upward incline (16).

fetus since the fetal lactate utilization rate (measured by tracer lactate experiments) exceeds the umbilical uptake of lactate. It is clear from the fetal hind limb studies that the carcass is a major site of net lactate production in the well-oxygenated fetus. Therefore, part of the lactate produced by fetal tissues is not oxidized at the site of production but is transported by the fetal circulation to other organs, such as the fetal liver, where it can then be utilized.

The hind limb of the fetus would appear to adapt to the fasting state in an analogous manner to that described for postnatal life; that is, the uptake of branch chain amino acids (leucine, isoleucine, and valine) is increased and the efflux of the gluconeogenic amino acids (glutamine and alanine) is also increased (22). Presumably, these compounds are then available to the fetal liver as carbon precursors for glucose synthesis. Interorgan cycling between the fetal hind limb and the fetal liver has also been described for acetate and lactate, the hind limb taking up acetate and releasing lactate, and conversely, the liver taking up lactate and releasing acetate (30).

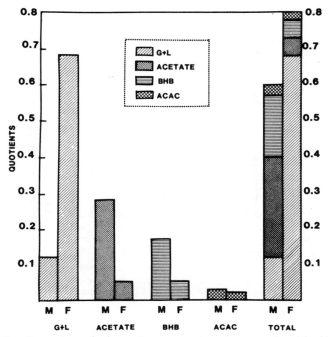

Figure 5-5: Comparison of substrate/oxygen quotients in maternal and fetal hind limbs. G + L, Glucose + lactate; BHB, β-hydroxybutyrate; ACAC, acetoacetate (30, 31).

FETAL LIVER METABOLISM

The liver is another fetal organ for which metabolic data have been collected. In 1976 Sparks *et al.* (32) reported a striking observation on isolated perfused fetal monkey livers. They found that there was no significant net uptake of glucose at any glucose concentration, whereas there was a net galactose uptake. Glycogen synthetase activity increased only in the presence of galactose, and its increase was most pronounced in the presence of galactose + insulin (Figure 5-6). Net glycogen accretion occurred only when fetal livers were perfused with galactose, and no net glycogen accretion occurred with glucose alone even in the face of high glucose concentrations and high insulin concentrations.

More recently, there has been considerable research in adult metabolism directed at the question of whether the glycogen accumulation in the liver postprandially is derived from glucose entering the portal circulation from the gastrointestinal tract or from three-carbon precursors such as lactate and alanine. A variety of approaches have been used to address

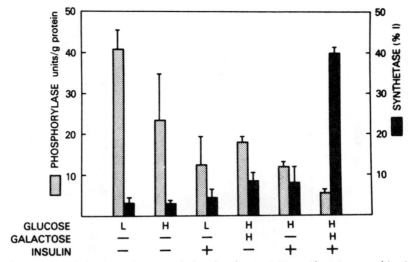

Figure 5-6: Glycogen synthetase and phosphorylase activities with various combinations of perfusate glucose, galactose, and insulin. Values shown are means ± SEM of synthetase and phosphorylase activity after 30 min of perfusion under conditions shown. For comparison, animals are grouped by presence (+) or absence (−) of insulin at 10^{-7} M and by glucose and galactose concentration. High concentrations (H) are between 275 and 400 mg/100 ml; lower concentrations (L) are between 100 and 250 mg/100 ml (32).

this question, and a clear answer is not yet forthcoming (19). However, it seems reasonably well established that most of the glucose taken in by the gastrointestinal tract is not accounted for by utilization by the gastrointestinal tract nor by net hepatic uptake. For example, Abumrad et al. (1) showed that only about 24% of an ingested glucose load could be accounted for by net hepatic uptake. From a perinatal biology viewpoint, it is interesting that approximately 20–25% of the ingested glucose load in their studies was consumed by the gastrointestinal tract in these adult dogs. This can be compared to the net glucose utilization by the placenta of the total glucose load delivered to the fetus. In both instances the organ of transport has a fairly high utilization rate of glucose reducing the total quantity of glucose delivered to the organism.

Levitsky et al. (21) reported that when [U-^{14}C]lactate infusion was given into the fetal circulation, they could identify no [^{14}C]glucose in the fetal circulation; however, fetal liver glycogen had a specific activity 3.3% of that in fetal plasma lactate. Sparks et al. (33) reported a net lactate and glucose uptake by the fetal liver in the well-nourished sheep. Thus, some of the placental lactate production and delivery into the umbilical circulation could be accounted for by the hepatic uptake. Furthermore, they demonstrated that if lactate is infused into the fetus fetal hepatic lactate uptake increases, and associated with this increase, the fetal liver has a net glucose output. These data suggest that liver glycogen accretion in the perinatal period may be derived from carbon sources other than glucose. In the neonatal period galactose may represent a principal carbon source. During *in utero* development other carbon compounds, such as glutamine, alanine, lactate, and pyruvate, may be the more important precursors.

In the newborn lamb a linear relationship between blood flow and oxygen consumption has been described for the liver (11). This is a surprising finding and needs further confirmation. It implies a marked susceptibility of metabolic rate in this organ to any redistribution of cardiac output. By contrast, in fetal lambs intestinal $\dot{V}_{O_2}$ only decreased with severe hypoxemia associated with a marked reduction in intestinal blood flow (10). Bristow *et al.* (4) reported an oxygen consumption rate for the fetal liver of 3.9 and 4.4 ml/100 g/min for the right and left lobes, respectively, or approximately 180 μmol/100 g/min, which is similar to the weight-specific oxygen consumption of the fetal brain. Given the large size of the liver, this represents approximately 20% of the total fetal oxygen requirements. These investigators demonstrated that there was no significant uptake of glucose by the liver, and under conditions of severe hypoxia there was a significant net efflux of glucose from the liver presumably from glycogenolysis.

CEREBRAL METABOLISM

The metabolism of the developing brain has been studied fairly extensively under both *in vitro* and *in vivo* conditions. In some respects the data collected under both sets of experimental conditions are in agreement, and in other areas they are not. To address first an area of controversy, *in vitro* studies had suggested that the immature brain may rely upon anaerobic glycolysis for its energy needs with glucose being metabolized extensively to lactate. In contrast, several *in vivo* studies have established that at least in fetal sheep brain there is no appreciable net production of lactate and that there is a relatively small change in the lactate : pyruvate ratio across the cerebral circulation (17). Furthermore, in the last month of gestation the brain of fetal lambs has been shown to have a high rate of oxygen consumption (i.e., 4.04 ± 0.17 ml/100 g/min) (17, 18, 35). While this is the only species in which the metabolic rate of the fetal brain has been measured under chronic steady-state conditions, the oxygen consumption rates of the brain of newborn baboons and newborn human infants have been estimated under acute conditions. The estimates were 2.5 ml/100 g/min in the baboon (20) and 2.3 ml/100 g/min in the newborn infants (26), both representing fairly high rates of oxygen consumption, although not as high as in the fetal lamb. Thus, all of the *in vivo* data support the conclusion that the developing brain derives its energy from aerobic metabolism. In postnatal life under normal fed state conditions, glucose is the main energy source for brain metabolism. Studies of metabolic quotients across the cerebral circulation of fetal lambs have established that under normal physiologic conditions the cerebral glucose/oxygen quotient is approximately 1.0. For example, in one study the average quotient was 0.99 with confidence limits between 0.92 and 1.06 (17). It is apparent from such data that glucose is the main substrate of cerebral metabolism in prenatal life as well.

In all mammals that have been studied, the fetal blood does not have high concentrations of ketoacids when the pregnant animal is in the fed state. However, in some species the placenta is quite permeable to ketoacids. Thus, during starvation or during a diabetic ketoacidosis when maternal arterial concentrations of ketoacids are elevated, fetal concentrations would also be elevated in those species. Therefore, it is appropriate to ask what is the impact of increased β-hydroxybutyrate or acetoacetate concentrations upon brain metabolism in fetal life. This question was given added clinical relevance by the suggestion that ketonuria in diabetic mothers may be causally related to retarded neurologic development in their infants (6, 34). Ketonuria in the mother would presumably reflect increased ketone body concentration in the maternal blood leading to increased delivery of ketone bodies to the fetus since it would appear that the human placenta is quite permeable to β-hydroxybutyrate and acetoacetate. Several interesting studies have been carried out on fetal brain under *in vitro* conditions that explore the effects of increasing ketoacid concentrations upon cerebral metabolism in the fetus or newborn. For example, DeVivo *et al.* (8) reported that in newborn rat brain [^{14}C]β-hydroxybutyrate differentially labeled brain glutamate, aspartate, and alanine in contrast to [^{14}C]glucose (Table 5-1). Although this study was carried out on newborn brain tissue, it is likely to apply to late fetal life as well. The activities of the three enzymes required for oxidation of ketoacids were shown to be present in brain tissue obtained from human fetuses of 32 weeks gestation. In a later report these observations were confirmed and extended to 8–10 weeks gestation (25). In these studies the carbon from ketoacids has been shown to be incorporated into cerebral proteins presumably through the incorporation into amino acids. In addition to incorporation into cerebral proteins, the carbon from the ketoacids is also used for lipid synthesis in the developing brain (24). In neonatal rat

Table 5-1

The Specific Activities of Certain Amino Acids in Brain Tissue of Newborn Rats Injected with [2-^{14}C]Glucose or [3-^{14}C]β-Hydroxybutyrate

[^{14}C] Precursor	n	Amino acid	Specific activity[a] (dpm[b]/μmol)	p value
[2-^{14}C]Glucose	6	Glutamate	1620 ± 150	$p < 0.001$
[3-^{14}C]β-OHB[c]	5	Glutamate	4290 ± 250	
[2-^{14}C]Glucose	6	Glutamine	480 ± 180	—
[3-^{14}C]β-OHB	5	Glutamine	630 ± 70	
[2-^{14}C]Glucose	6	Aspartate	1200 ± 310	$p < 0.10$
[3-^{14}C]β-OHB	5	Aspartate	1960 ± 130	
[2-^{14}C]Glucose	6	Alanine	2180 ± 320	$p < 0.001$
[3-^{14}C]β-OHB	5	Alanine	115 ± 37	
[2-^{14}C]Glucose	6	GABA	48 ± 27	—
[3-^{14}C]β-OHB	5	GABA	435 ± 74	

[a] Values are given as mean ± SEM.
[b] dpm = disintegration per minute.
[c] β-OHB, β-hydroxybutyrate.

brain under *in vitro* conditions, the ketoacids are better precursors than glucose for lipid synthesis. Considering the concern of a possible link between maternal ketoacidosis and fetal brain growth, the report of Bhasin and Shambaugh (2) of an inhibitory effect of ketoacids upon pyrimidine biosynthesis in fetal rat brain may be relevant. Figure 5-7 from their report illustrates the progressive inhibition of uridine synthesis by increasing β-hydroxybutyrate concentrations. The evidence that fetal brain can oxidize ketones has been reviewed by Shambaugh *et al.* (27, 29). They have shown that fetal brain slices will decrease their oxidation of other fuels such as glucose when incubated with high concentrations of ketones (28).

Studies directed at rates of protein synthesis within the brain describe a pattern similar to that of the whole body; namely, that the high rates of protein synthesis in early life are accompanied by high rates of protein degradation. In one study by Dunlop *et al.* (9) on neonatal rat brain, the degradation rate was 65% of the synthetic rate. Figure 5-8 from this study of Dunlop *et al.* (9) illustrates the changes in protein synthetic rate, degradation rate, and net protein accretion rate at different stages of postnatal development in the rat. Of course, these developmental patterns will be different in different species depending upon the maturity of the brain at the time of delivery. It is important to note that variations in the energy requirements for synthetic processes are likely to combine with variations

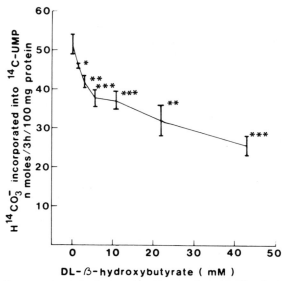

Figure 5-7: Concentrations of β-hydroxybutyrate are plotted on the abscissa and H^{14}CO$_3^-$ incorporation into [^{14}C]uridine monophosphate ([^{14}C]UMP) is shown on the ordinate. Mean ± 1 SEM (bars) is given. Statistical significance of each value when compared to data obtained in absence of β-hydroxybutyrate is shown by asterisks: *, $p < 0.05$; **, $p < 0.01$; ***, $p < 0.001$ (2).

in requirements for establishing and maintaining ion gradients to produce large changes in the rate of oxidative metabolism of neural tissues during development. It is possible, for example, that in early developmental stages synthetic processes dominate over ion transport in determining oxygen requirements and that the opposite is true at later stages. Thus, as the process of building new structures declines in importance and complex neural interactions become functional, different regions of the brain may go through a sequence of maximal and minimal energy requirements that underlie temporal and regional variations in their vulnerability to hypoxic damage. For these reasons, one must be careful in drawing inferences from the current meager knowledge of fetal cerebral metabolism. On the one hand, the notion that fetal cerebral tissues depend on oxidative metabolism that is fueled preferentially by glucose is likely to be generally valid. On the other hand, measurements of oxygen consumption rate at one stage of gestation and in one species are probably not representative of oxygen consumption rates at other stages and in other species. The problem of estimating the cerebral oxygen requirement of the human fetus at term illustrates some of the difficulties involved. If we

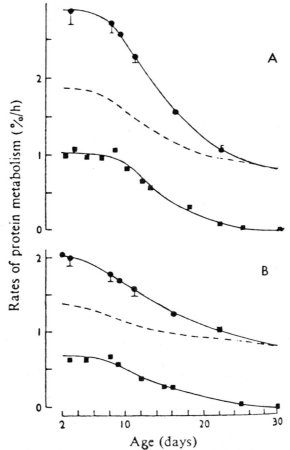

Figure 5-8: Rates of protein metabolism at different stages of development for the cerebellum (A) and cerebral hemisphere (B). Rates of synthesis and accretion were determined as stated in the text (9). The rate of degradation is the difference between the synthesis and accretion rates. ●, protein synthesis rate; ■, protein accretion rate; ---, protein degradation rate (9). Reprinted by permission from *Biochemistry Journal*, vol. 170, pp. 637–642, copyright © 1978 The Biochemical Society, London.

were to attribute to the human fetal brain the weight-specific oxygen consumption of the fetal lamb brain, the estimated oxygen consumption rate would be very high, approximately 15 ml_{STP}/min, because the cerebral mass is approximately seven times greater in the human than in the ovine term fetus. A more conservative estimate (approximately 9 ml_{STP}/min) is arrived at if we attribute to the term human fetus the estimated cerebral oxygen requirements of the human newborn. Since both estimates have serious limitations, we are missing a crucial bit of quantitative information about the energy and circulatory needs of the fetal brain in humans.

There have been studies attempting to describe the changes in permeability of the blood brain barrier at different developmental stages. Cornford et al. (7) reported studies carried out on newborn and adult rabbits. Using compounds with a wide range of lipid solubilities, they found that newborn and adult brains were very similar in their relationship between lipid solubility and cerebral penetrability of the various compounds. Whether this is true during fetal life has not yet been investigated.

CARDIAC METABOLISM

The metabolic requirements of the adult heart are fairly similar among mammals. Glucose is not the primary energy source, although it is taken up by the heart to some extent. Free fatty acids and amino acids are the most important fuels for the adult heart (23).

The metabolic characteristics of the heart change quite markedly during development. Studies by Foa et al. (14) in 1965 upon the embryonic chick heart illustrated the fact that at 5 days of age glucose uptake was independent of insulin (Figure 5-9). In contrast, at the same stage, insulin stimulates the incorporation of [^{14}C]acetate into lipids. An important contribution in pinpointing some of the differences of cardiac metabolism in early development versus later in life came in the report by Wittels and Bressler in 1965 (37). Working with homogenates of newborn rat hearts, they demonstrated that the oxidation rate of [^{14}C]palmitate was only 20% of that of adult hearts and was associated with low carnitine acyl CoA transferase activity and a greater capacity for glucose oxidation. This was extended to newborn dogs by Breuer et al. (3) who demonstrated that in the neonatal period there was no significant extraction of long chain free fatty acids from the coronary circulation coupled with a large glucose extraction.

These basic observations of a dependence upon carbohydrates as an energy source for the developing heart in contrast to the oxidation of fatty acids in adult hearts were extended to two other species. Werner et al. (36), working with perfused newborn piglet hearts, demonstrated the reliance upon carbohydrates to sustain energy levels as well as arterial pressure and ventricular outputs. In addition, they found that the carbohydrates were used for aerobic oxidation and that glycolysis was not a major pathway for energy production as shown by a minimal lactate production rate.

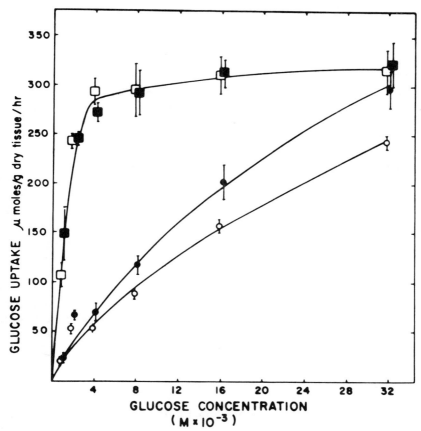

Figure 5-9: Effect of initial glucose concentration in incubation medium on glucose uptake by chick embryo hearts. Five-day-old hearts with (■) or without (□) insulin; nine-day-old hearts with (●) or without (○) insulin. Insulin concentration is 0.01 U/ml. Each point represents means ± SE of five experiments (14).

Observations by Fisher *et al.* (12, 13) in fetal lambs studied under chronic steady-state conditions showed a large net lactate uptake by the coronary circulation demonstrating that the fetal lamb heart in contrast to skeletal muscle (see hind limb metabolism) is a net consumer of lactate under normal well-oxygenated conditions, not a net producer. Furthermore, the sum of the glucose + lactate + pyruvate/oxygen quotients, representing the total carbohydrate uptake that was measured in those studies, was equal to 0.97; that is, virtually all of the oxygen uptake could be accounted for by the uptake of carbohydrates.

The findings regarding lactate consumption by the heart of newborn piglets and fetal lambs are important because there had been the supposition that glycolysis might play an important role in meeting the energy demands of the developing heart. The oxygen consumption of the newborn piglet and fetal lamb hearts, while studied under different conditions, are in fairly good agreement. The oxygen consumption of the isolated perfused piglet heart was approximately 260–430 mmol/100 g wet weight/min and that of the lamb approximately 382 mmol/100 g/min.

Under conditions of a moderate reduction in fetal arterial P_{O_2}, insufficient to produce fetal acidosis, there are no significant changes in myocardial oxygen or substrate uptakes. Comparable studies have not been carried out under hypoxic conditions sufficient to produce a metabolic acidosis or a significant reduction in fetal oxygen consumption.

The studies in several species demonstrating the dependence of the developing heart upon carbohydrate consumption are particularly relevant when considered against the background of the clinical reports describing cardiac failure in hypoglycemic newborn infants without evidence of congenital heart disease. Furthermore, while some of the cardiomyopathy of the infants of diabetic mothers undoubtedly contributes to the myocardial dysfunction commonly found in these babies, hypoglycemic episodes may also contribute. It is not yet known at what developmental stages the human heart becomes primarily dependent upon the oxidation of free fatty acids.

OTHER ORGANS

There are less data for other fetal organs. The oxygen consumption rate of the fetal intestine has been measured under chronic steady-state conditions both in normoxic and hypoxic fetal lambs (5). The oxygen consumption is low compared with that of other fetal organs, approximately 2.1 ml/100 g/min or 94 μmoles/100 g/min. A significant uptake of glucose, α-amino nitrogen and lactate across the gastrointestinal tract has been found in chronically catheterized fetal lambs (5). The lactate uptake was appreciable despite the relatively small size and lower metabolic rate of the gut representing 13% of the umbilical uptake. More recently, the oxygen glucose and lactate consumption of the fetal kidney have been reported (15). While the rates are very low, a net glucose efflux from the kidney was found coincident with a net oxygen and lactate uptake. Only 42% of the renal oxygen consumption was accounted for by net carbohydrate uptake implying significant utilization of other substrates for oxidative metabolism.

REFERENCES

1. Abumrad, N.N., Cherrington, A.D., Williams, P.E., Lacy, W.W. and Rabin, D. (1982). *Absorption and disposition of a glucose load in the conscious dog.* American Journal of Physiology **242**, E398-E406.
2. Bhasin, S. and Shambaugh, G.E. III (1982). *Fetal fuels. V. Ketone bodies inhibit pyrimidine biosynthesis in fetal rat brain.* American Journal of Physiology **243**, E234-E239.
3. Breuer, E., Barta, E., Zlatos, L. and Pappova, E. (1968). *Developmental changes of myocardial metabolism. II. Myocardial metabolism of fatty acids in the early postnatal period in dogs.* Biology of the Neonate **12**, 54–64.
4. Bristow, J., Rudolph, A.M., Itskovitz, J. and Barnes, R. (1983). *Hepatic oxygen and glucose metabolism in the fetal lamb. Response to hypoxia.* Journal of Clinical Investigation **71**, 1047–1061.
5. Charlton, V.E., Reis, B.L. and Lofgren, D.J. (1979). *Consumption of carbohydrates, amino acids and oxygen across the intestinal circulation in the fetal sheep.* Journal of Developmental Physiology **1**, 329–336.
6. Churchill, J.A., Berendes, H.W. and Nemore, J. (1969). *Neuropsychological deficits in children of diabetic mothers: a report from the collaborative study of cerebral palsy.* American Journal of Obstetrics and Gynecology **105**, 257–268.
7. Cornford, E.M., Braun, L.D., Oldendorf, W.H. and Hill, M.A. (1982). *Comparison of lipid-mediated blood-brain-barrier penetrability in neonates and adults.* American Journal of Physiology **243**, C161-C168.
8. DeVivo, D.C., Leckie, M.P. and Agrawal, H.C. (1973). *The differential incorporation of beta-hydroxybutyrate and glucose into brain glutamate in the newborn rat.* Brain Research **55**, 485–490.
9. Dunlop, D.S., van Elden, W. and Lajtha, A. (1978). *Protein degradation rates in regions of the central nervous system in vivo during development.* Biochemistry Journal **170**, 637–642.
10. Edelstone, D.I. and Holzman, I.R. (1982). *Fetal intestinal oxygen consumption at various levels of oxygenation.* American Journal of Physiology **242**, H50-H54.
11. Edelstone, D.I., Paulone, M.E. and Holzman, I.R. (1984). *Hepatic oxygenation during arterial hypoxemia in neonatal lambs.* American Journal of Obstetrics and Gynecology **150**, 513–518.
12. Fisher, D.J., Heymann, M.A. and Rudolph, A.M. (1980). *Myocardial oxygen and carbohydrate consumption in fetal lambs in utero and in adult sheep.* American Journal of Physiology **238**, H399-H405.
13. Fisher, D.J., Heymann, M.A. and Rudolph, A.M. (1982). *Fetal myocardial oxygen and carbohydrate consumption during acutely induced hypoxemia.* American Journal of Physiology **242**, H657-H661.
14. Foa, P.P., Melli, M., Berger, C.K., Billinger, D. and Guidotti, G.G. (1965). *Action of insulin on chick embryo heart.* Federation Proceedings **24**, 1046–1050.
15. Iwamoto, H.S. and Rudolph, A.M. (1983). *Chronic renal venous catheterization in fetal sheep.* American Journal of Physiology **245**, H524-H527.
16. Jarrett, I.G., Filsell, O.H. and Ballard, F.J. (1976). *Utilization of oxidizable substrate by the sheep hindlimb, effects of starvation and exercise.* Metabolism **25**, 523–531.
17. Jones, M.D. Jr., Burd, L.I., Makowski, E.L., Meschia, G. and Battaglia, F.C. (1975). *Cerebral metabolism in sheep: a comparative study of the adult, the lamb, and the fetus.* American Journal of Physiology **229**, 235–239.

18. Jones, M.D. Jr., Traystman, R.J., Simmons, M.A. and Molteni, R.A. (1981). *Effects of changes in arterial O_2 content on cerebral blood flow in the lamb.* American Journal of Physiology **240**, H209-H215.
19. Katz, J. and McGarry, J.D. (1984). *The glucose paradox: Is glucose a substrate for liver metabolism?* Journal of Clinical Investigation **74**, 1901-1909.
20. Levitsky, L.L., Fisher, D.E., Paton, J.B. and DeLannoy, C.W. (1977). *Fasting plasma levels of glucose, acetoacetate, D-β-hydroxybutyrate, glycerol, and lactate in the baboon infant: correlation with cerebral uptake of substrates and oxygen.* Pediatric Research **11**, 298-302.
21. Levitsky, L.L., Paton, J.B. and Fisher, D.E. (1985). *Lactate is a glycogenic precursor in the ovine fetus.* Pediatric Research **19**, 315A (abstract).
22. Liechty, E.A. and Lemons, J.A. (1984). *Changes in ovine fetal hindlimb amino acid metabolism during maternal fasting.* American Journal of Physiology **246**, E430-E435.
23. Most, A.S., Brachfeld, N., Gorlin, R. and Wahren, J. (1969). *Free fatty acid metabolism of the human heart at rest.* Journal of Clinical Investigation **48**, 1177-1188.
24. Patel, M.S. and Owen, O.E. (1977). *Development and regulation of lipid synthesis from ketone bodies by rat brain.* Journal of Neurochemistry **28**, 109-114.
25. Patel, M.S., Johnson, C.A., Rajan, R. and Owen, O.E. (1975). *The metabolism of ketone bodies in developing human brain: Development of ketone-body-utilizing enzymes and ketone bodies as precursors for lipid synthesis.* Journal of Neurochemistry **25**, 905-908.
26. Settergren, G., Lindblad, B.S. and Persson, B. (1976). *Cerebral blood flow and exchange of oxygen, glucose, ketone bodies, lactate, pyruvate and amino acids in infants.* Acta Paediatrica Scandinavia **65**, 343-353.
27. Shambaugh, G.E. III. (1985). *Ketone body metabolism in the mother and fetus.* Federation Proceedings **44**, 2347-2351.
28. Shambaugh, G.E. III, Koehler, R.A. and Freinkel, N. (1977). *Fetal fuels. II. Contributions of selected carbon fuels to oxidative metabolism in the rat conceptus.* American Journal of Physiology **233**, E457-E461.
29. Shambaugh, G.E. III, Mrozak, S.C. and Freinkel, N. (1977). *Fetal fuels. I. Utilization of ketones by isolated tissues at various stages of maturation and maternal nutrition during late gestation.* Metabolism **26**, 623-636.
30. Singh, S., Sparks, J., Hay, W.W. Jr., Battaglia, F.C. and Meschia, G. (1983). *Acetate metabolism in the maternal and fetal hindlimb, uteroplacenta, and fetal liver of the sheep.* In "Thirtieth Annual Meeting of the Society for Gynecologic Investigation," Scientific Program and Abstracts, pp 276.
31. Singh, S., Sparks, J.W., Meschia, G., Battaglia, F.C. and Makowski, E.L. (1984). *Comparison of fetal and maternal hind limb metabolic quotients in sheep.* American Journal of Obstetrics and Gynecology **149**, 441-449.
32. Sparks, J.W., Lynch, A., Chez, R.A. and Glinsmann, W.H. (1976). *Glycogen regulation in isolated perfused near term monkey liver.* Pediatric Research **10**, 51-56.
33. Sparks, J.W., Hay, W.W. Jr., Meschia, G. and Battaglia, F.C. (1985). *Lactic acid tolerance in the non-hypoxic fetal lamb.* Pediatric Research (Suppl.) **19**, 1263, (abstract).
34. Stehbens, J.A., Baker, G.L. and Kitchell, M. (1977). *Outcome of ages 1, 3, and 5 years of children born to diabetic women.* American Journal of Obstetrics and Gynecology **127**, 408-413.
35. Tsoulos, N.G., Schneider, J.M., Colwill, J.R., Meschia, G., Makowski, E.L. and Bat-

taglia, F.C. (1972). *Cerebral glucose utilization during aerobic metabolism in fetal sheep*. Pediatric Research **6**, 182–186.

36. Werner, J.C., Whitman, V., Fripp, R.R., Schuler, H.G., Musselman, J. and Sham, R.L. (1983). *Fatty acid and glucose utilization in isolated, working fetal pig hearts*. American Journal of Physiology **245**, E19-E23.

37. Wittels, B. and Bressler, R. (1965). *Lipid metabolism in the newborn heart*. Journal of Clinical Investigation **44**, 1639–1646.

6

Fetal Respiratory Physiology

GENERAL CONSIDERATIONS

The transport of oxygen from the atmosphere to fetal tissues can be visualized as a sequence of steps which alternate bulk transport with transport by diffusion (28). These steps require a progressive decrease of oxygen pressure along the transport route (Figure 6-1). Oxygen is transported from atmosphere to alveoli by action of the respiratory muscles that ventilate the lungs (step 1) and then diffuses from alveolar air into maternal blood (step 2). Maternal arterial blood, propelled by the action of the maternal heart, transports oxygen from the lungs to the placenta (step 3). In the placenta, oxygen molecules diffuse from maternal to fetal blood (step 4). The oxygenated blood returning from the placenta to the fetus commingles within the fetal body with less oxygenated blood (step 5) to form the blood that perfuses the fetal organs (step 6). In the final step, oxygen diffuses from fetal blood to the cells of the fetal tissues, down the P_{O_2} gradient created and maintained by the metabolic activity of these cells. The transport of CO_2 from fetal tissues to atmosphere follows the oxygen route in reverse, each step being accompanied by a decrease of P_{CO_2} (Figure 6-1).

Both maternal and fetal blood transport oxygen in two forms: free (that is, physically dissolved in blood) and bound to hemoglobin. In any blood sample these two forms are in reversible equilibrium. The nomenclature which is used to identify different aspects of this equilibrium is summa-

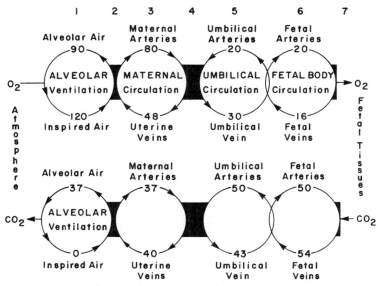

Figure 6-1: Diagram showing the decrement of P_{O_2} as oxygen is transported from atmosphere to fetus, and the decrement of P_{CO_2} as CO_2 is transported from fetus to atmosphere. Representative values (Torr) of P_{O_2} and P_{CO_2} are given for pregnant sheep at 1500 m altitude.

rized in Table 6-1. From the table one can see that each variable can either be measured directly or calculated from other measurements.

In contrast to this broad overview, it is not possible to give a detailed description of fetal respiratory physiology without taking into account important species differences. For this reason we shall first analyze the respiratory physiology of the fetal sheep, about which there are ample and reliable data, and then consider comparative aspects in other species.

OXYGEN TRANSPORT ACROSS THE OVINE PLACENTA

As an introduction to the respiratory function of the ovine placenta, consider the numerical data of Figure 6-2, which are an example of normal physiologic conditions in the last month of pregnancy. The gravid uterus, carrying a 3-kg fetus, is perfused by maternal blood at the rate of 1200 ml/min. Approximately 1000 ml/min of blood (83% of uterine blood flow) perfuses the placental cotyledons, another 160 ml/min perfuses the endometrium, and 40 ml/min perfuses the myometrium. On the other side of the placental barrier, the fetus pumps through the umbilical arteries

Table 6-1

Blood Oxygen Transport: Nomenclature, Symbols,
Units, Measuring Instruments, and Interrelationships

Nomenclature	Symbol	Units	Basic measuring instruments
Free O_2	$(O_2)_F$	mM [a]	—
O_2 bound to hemoglobin	HbO_2	mM	—
O_2 content	O_2	mM	E.g., Van Slyke apparatus, gas chromatograph
O_2 pressure	P_{O_2}	mm Hg [b]	P_{O_2} electrode
Hemoglobin	Hb	mM	Spectrophotometer
O_2 capacity	O_2 CAP	mM	—
O_2 saturation	S	%	Spectrophotometer
P_{O_2} at S = 50%	P_{50}	mmHg	—

Interrelationships

$$S = HbO_2/O_2 \text{ CAP}$$
$$O_2 \text{ CAP} = 4Hb = O_2 \text{ carried by Hb when S} = 100\% \text{ [c]}$$
$$O_2 = HbO_2 + (O_2)_F = S \times (O_2 \text{ CAP}) + (O_2)_F$$
$$(O_2)_F = \alpha_{O_2} P_{O_2} \text{ (where } \alpha_{O_2} = O_2 \text{ solubility coefficient)}$$

[a] Millimoles per liter of blood. Another unit used often in reporting the O_2 content of blood is volume percent, i.e., ml_{STP} of O_2 per dl of blood (1 mM = 2.24 vol %).

[b] The millimeter of mercury unit (mm Hg) can also be called a Torr. Another unit of pressure used frequently in the literature is the pascal (Pa) (1 Torr = 133.3 Pa).

[c] Each hemoglobin molecule can combine with four molecules of O_2. Oxygen capacity can be calculated also by measuring the O_2 content of blood exposed to a high P_{O_2} that fully saturates Hb with O_2 and by subtracting from the measured value the concentration of free O_2.

600 ml/min. Approximately 93% of the umbilical blood flow perfuses the cotyledons and 7% perfuses the intercotyledonary chorion in contact with the surface of the endometrial mucosa. Maternal blood with oxygen capacity 6.4 mM enters the uterine circulation with P_{O_2} at 80 Torr and oxygen saturation at 90% and exits via the uterine veins with P_{O_2} at 50 Torr and 69% saturated. By application of the Fick principle one can calculate the amount of oxygen taken up by the pregnant uterus to be 1.6 mM/min. Fetal blood with an oxygen capacity 6.8 mM enters the umbilical circulation via the umbilical arteries with P_{O_2} at 24 Torr and 55% saturated and exits the umbilical circulation via the umbilical vein with P_{O_2} at 32 Torr and 80% saturated. Thus, one can calculate the net amount of oxygen flowing from placenta to fetus to be 1.0 mM/min.

The reason for introducing placental oxygen transfer by way of a numerical example is that the most interesting aspects of this physiologic process are quantitative. The extremely low P_{O_2} of fetal blood is of outstanding interest in this regard. This low P_{O_2} is the result of several condi-

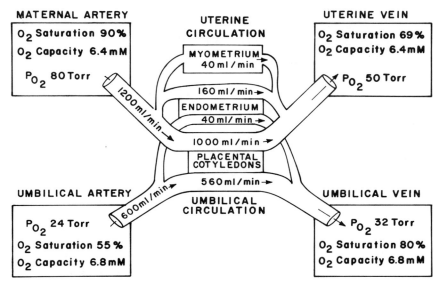

Figure 6-2: Numerical data that demonstrate normal conditions of placental oxygen transfer in sheep.

tions that hinder fetal oxygenation, and it requires unique fetal adaptive mechanisms.

HINDRANCES TO FETAL OXYGENATION

As discussed in Chapter 2, an important property of the ovine placenta is that the uterine and umbilical circulations form an "imperfect venous equilibrator." The umbilical venous concentration of molecules diffusing from mother to fetus is less than the uterine venous concentration, even under conditions of flow-limited diffusion. This knowledge implies that umbilical venous P_{O_2} cannot be as high as uterine venous P_{O_2} even under conditions that favor the equilibration of maternal and fetal blood P_{O_2} within the placental capillaries. Direct experimental evidence has verified this implication (39). One hundred percent oxygen was administered to pregnant ewes to elevate the P_{O_2} gradient between maternal and fetal arterial blood and to promote the rapid equilibration of P_{O_2} across the placental barrier. In addition, the oxyhemoglobin dissociation curve of maternal blood was shifted to the right by inducing a state of maternal metabolic acidosis with the infusion of ammonium chloride. In each experiment, umbilical venous P_{O_2} remained substantially less than uterine venous P_{O_2} (Figure 6-3).

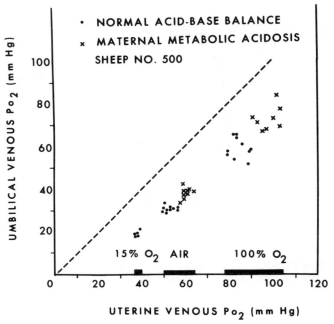

Figure 6-3: Relationship of umbilical venous P_{O_2} to uterine venous P_{O_2} in a pregnant sheep. The dashed line is the line of identity (39).

A second placental property which hinders fetal oxygenation is its high oxygen consumption rate. (In the representative example of Figure 6-2, fetal oxygen uptake is only 62% of uterine oxygen uptake.) The high metabolic rate of the placenta was discussed in Chapter 3.

The above two factors have been confirmed experimentally. Theoretically there is a third factor which may hinder fetal oxygenation: the placental oxygen diffusing capacity (D_p). In theory it could be inadequate for complete equilibration of maternal and fetal blood P_{O_2} across the placental barrier. However, the importance of D_p in limiting fetal oxygenation is not clear. There are several reasons for this uncertainty. Placental oxygen diffusing capacity is usually defined as the ratio of oxygen transfer to the fetus from the placenta (R_{O_2}) over the mean P_{O_2} difference ($\overline{\Delta P_{O_2}}$) between maternal and fetal red cells within the placenta:

$$D_p = R_{O_2}/\overline{\Delta P_{O_2}} \tag{6-1}$$

Thus defined, placental oxygen diffusing capacity becomes a function of several factors: the placental permeability to oxygen molecules, the rate of dissociation of maternal oxyhemoglobin, and the rate of association of

PARTIAL PRESSURE
DIFFERENCE

DIFFUSION
RESISTANCE

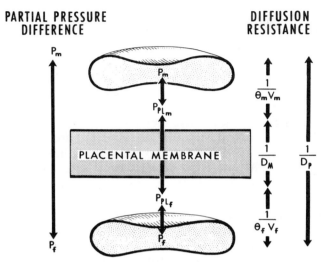

Figure 6-4: Schematic representation of the maternal to fetal partial pressure differences and resistances to diffusion of oxygen. The total P_{O_2} difference $(P_m - P_f)$ consists of (1) the difference from the interior of the maternal red cell to plasma $(P_m - P_{pl,m})$; (2) the difference across the membrane from maternal to fetal plasma $(P_{pl,m} - P_{pl,f})$; and (3) the difference from fetal plasma to the interior of the fetal erythrocyte $(P_{pl,f} - P_f)$. The total resistance to diffusion $(1/D_p)$ is the sum of the individual resistances: (1) the resistance of maternal blood $(1/\theta_m V_m)$; (2) the placental membrane resistance $(1/D_M)$; and (3) the resistance of fetal blood $(1/\theta_f V_f)$. The θ_m and θ_f factors represent primarily the rates of reaction of maternal and fetal hemoglobin with oxygen. V_m and V_f are the volumes of blood in maternal and fetal placental exchange vessels (25).

oxygen with fetal hemoglobin (Figure 6-4). It also depends upon the placental oxygen consumption rate. The higher the rate of placental oxygen consumption, the lower the amount of oxygen transferred to the fetus for any given value of $\overline{\Delta P_{O_2}}$ (see the discussion on placental glucose transfer in Chapter 3 for reference to an analogous situation). Thus, Equation 6-1 should be rewritten to include the impact of uteroplacental oxygen consumption on the calculation of D_p:

$$D_p = (R_{O_2} + r_{O_2})/\overline{\Delta P_{O_2}} \qquad (6\text{-}2)$$

where r_{O_2} represents the portion of uteroplacental oxygen consumption which should be added to R_{O_2} to obviate the pitfall of making placental oxygen diffusing capacity dependent upon placental oxygen consumption. Unfortunately, the exact value of this correction is unknown. In any case, one of the major problems with addressing placental D_p has not been its definition but the seemingly impossible task of making an accurate estimate of $\overline{\Delta P_{O_2}}$. To circumvent this difficulty, Longo *et al.* (24, 25) measured the placental diffusing capacity for carbon monoxide and inferred placental D_p from it. The method for measuring CO diffusing capacity relies on the high affinity of hemoglobin for CO. Maternal hemoglobin which has been loaded with CO releases this gas slowly to fetal hemoglobin, so that an equilibrium between maternal and fetal blood is not attained for hours. Therefore, the mean concentration of carbonmonoxihemoglobin (HbCO) in maternal and fetal placental blood can be measured with precision because there is virtually no arteriovenous difference of HbCO across the uterine and umbilical circulations. However, despite the absence of HbCO arteriovenous differences, there is a relatively large P_{CO} difference across the uterine circulation (Figure 6-5), which is due to the effect of P_{O_2} on the equilibrium between CO and hemoglobin (24). This difference creates uncertainty in the estimation of the mean transplacental P_{CO} gradient and therefore in the estimation of CO diffusing capacity. Once this capacity is estimated, it is possible to estimate D_p from the solubility, molecular weight, and hemoglobin reaction rates of the CO and oxygen molecules (24, 25). According to such estimates the D_p of the ovine placenta is approximately 0.68 ml$_{STP}$/Torr/

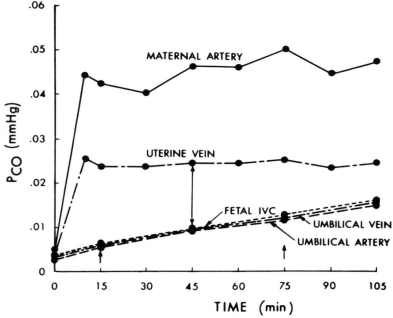

Figure 6-5: Partial pressure of carbon monoxide in the maternal and fetal blood vessels of sheep during maternal inhalation of CO (24).

kg/min (24). Hence, for a fetal oxygen uptake of 7 ml/kg/min the $\overline{\Delta P_{O_2}}$ calculated according to Equation 6-1 is approximately 10 Torr. The real value of $\overline{\Delta P_{O_2}}$ will be higher due to placental oxygen consumption. Another major problem is that inferences derived from estimates of placental D_p and $\overline{\Delta P_{O_2}}$ are model dependent. Calculations based on a concurrent flow model of placental exchange (Chapter 2, Figure 2-2) indicate that a D_p equal to 0.68 ml_{STP}/Torr/kg/min is sufficient for virtually complete equilibration of maternal and fetal venous P_{O_2} (23). If we were to assume, however, a placental model similar to the double pool model (Chapter 2, Figure 2-1) we would conclude that a sizable fraction (approximately half) of the uterine venous minus umbilical venous P_{O_2} difference is due to a low oxygen diffusing capacity, even though both models are venous equilibrators. Therefore, it is not yet clear whether placental diffusing capacity is a limiting factor that contributes significantly to the low P_{O_2} of fetal blood under normal physiologic conditions.

An important consequence of the complex anatomy of fetal circulation is that all regions of the fetal body are perfused by blood which is formed by mixing the blood returning from the placenta with less oxygenated blood returning from the fetal tissues. The only exception is the left lobe of the liver which is perfused almost exclusively by umbilical venous blood. The fetal circulation can be divided into three distinct sets of arteries in order of decreasing oxygen content and P_{O_2}: (a) the arteries that originate from the aorta above the *ductus arteriosus* carrying blood ejected by the left ventricle, (b) the arteries that originate below the *ductus arteriosus* carrying blood formed by the confluence of blood ejected by both the right and left ventricles, and (c) the pulmonary arteries that carry blood ejected from the right ventricle. Under normal physiologic conditions the oxygen content of blood in the ascending aorta is approximately 0.4 mM higher than in the abdominal aorta and approximately 0.7 mM higher than in the pulmonary artery (41). These differences in oxygen content are associated with differences in oxygen saturation and P_{O_2}. However, the P_{O_2} differences are relatively small because the high oxygen affinity of fetal blood tends to "buffer" the P_{O_2} of unsaturated fetal blood (Figure 6-6).

In summary, there are three major factors responsible for the low P_{O_2} of ovine fetal arterial blood:

1. The placenta functions as an imperfect venous equilibrator of the uterine and umbilical circulations.
2. The placenta has a high rate of oxygen consumption.
3. Fetal arterial blood is formed by mixing umbilical venous blood with less oxygenated blood.

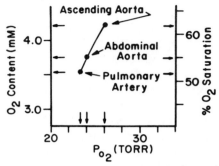

Figure 6-6: Differences in oxygen content, oxygen saturation, and P_{O_2} in the fetal arterial system.

In addition to the above factors, it is possible that the oxygen diffusing capacity of the placenta is insufficiently large to permit full equilibration of maternal and fetal blood P_{O_2} within each placental exchange unit.

MATERNAL FACTORS FAVORING FETAL OXYGENATION

The adverse effect on fetal oxygenation of an inefficient pattern of placental perfusion, a high rate of placental oxygen consumption, and the anatomical arrangement of the fetal circulation are compensated for by maternal and fetal adaptations that allow for an adequate oxygen supply to fetal tissues.

The principal maternal adaptation is a high rate of uterine perfusion that maintains uterine venous P_{O_2} at a relatively high level. In late gestation in the sheep, the amount of uterine blood flow is twice the umbilical blood flow (Table 6-2) and represents approximately 15% of maternal cardiac output (Chapter 8).

Table 6-2

Simultaneously Measured Uterine and Umbilical Blood Flows in 17 Sheep, Each Carrying a Single Fetus[a]

	Fetal weight (kg)	Uterine blood flow (ml/min)	Umbilical blood flow (ml/min)	Uterine flow/ umbilical flow
	4.53	1598	812	1.97
($\pm$ SEM)	($\pm$ 0.26)	($\pm$ 92)	($\pm$ 63)	

[a] From Meschia *et al.* (31).

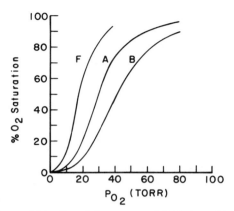

Figure 6-7: Oxyhemoglobin dissociation curves of fetal sheep blood (F), of adult sheep blood with ovine hemoglobin (A), and of adult sheep blood with ovine hemoglobin (B). The curves are representative of normal *in vivo* conditions.

At sea level or moderate altitudes, a low affinity of maternal hemoglobin for oxygen would favor fetal oxygenation by increasing the P_{O_2} of placental venous blood. There is no evidence that pregnancy induces physiologically significant changes in the oxygen affinity of maternal blood. However, the requirements of fetal oxygenation may act as a selective pressure in decreasing the oxygen affinity of maternal hemoglobin. In this context it is interesting to note that adult sheep have two types of hemoglobin (hemoglobin A and B) with markedly different oxygen affinities (Figure 6-7). Ordinarily, animals homozygote for A and B hemoglobin coexist in the same flock, although at quite different frequencies in different breeds and locations. The sheep that provided data for Figure 6-2 were homozygote for the low affinity B type. A comparison of reproductive performance has shown that the homozygote B carriers have a higher incidence of multiple births than the homozygote A carriers (15). Whether this observation correlates with differences in fetal oxygenation is not known because there have been no systematic studies comparing fetuses of A and B carriers.

FETAL ADAPTATION TO LOW OXYGEN TENSION

The fetal adaptation to the low P_{O_2} of fetal blood has two major components: (a) production of red cells that contain hemoglobin with high oxygen affinity (Figure 6-7) and (b) a cardiac output that is high in relation to oxygen demands (Chapter 7). Note that the concept that these two aspects of fetal physiology "adapt" the fetus to the low P_{O_2} environment created by the placenta does not imply that they developed in response to placentation. Avian and amphibian embryos also have red cells with high oxygen affinity, suggesting an independent origin of the fetal adaptation (32).

The advantage of producing red cells with high oxygen affinity is that under normal physiologic conditions each cell circulating through the placenta returns to the fetal body almost fully saturated with oxygen. In other words, for any given fetal hematocrit, high oxygen affinity tends to maximize the amount of oxygen carried by fetal blood. Although of vital importance, this biochemical adaptation increases only the oxygen saturation and oxygen contents of fetal blood; it does not increase the P_{O_2} of fetal blood. In fact, it contributes in making fetal P_{O_2} lower than it might otherwise be. To understand why this is so, we must contrast two models of placental perfusion, one represented by a venous equilibrator with even perfusion and the other by a venous equilibrator composed of exchange units each having different maternal : fetal perfusion ratios (30). In both models we assume P_{O_2} equilibration at the venous end of each exchanger. In the first model, umbilical venous P_{O_2} is not dependent on the position of the fetal oxyhemoglobin dissociation curve. If the oxyhemoglobin dissociation curve is shifted either to the left or to the right, umbilical venous P_{O_2} remains constant while oxygen saturation changes (i.e., it increases with a shift to the left and decreases with a shift to the right). In the second model, which is more realistic, umbilical venous blood results from the mixing of blood streams with different oxygen saturations. Because of the nonlinearity of the oxyhemoglobin dissociate curve, mixing streams with different saturations yields a P_{O_2} in the collecting vein which is biased toward the low P_{O_2} values in the mixture. The bias is large if some of the streams are highly saturated and relatively

Table 6-3

**Oxygenation and pH of Umbilical Venous Blood
Before and After Exchange Transfusion of Adult
Sheep Blood (Hemoglobin Type B) in Fetal Lambs**[a,b]

	Before transfusion	After transfusion
O_2 saturation (%)	79.1	51.3
O_2 capacity (mM)	6.8	6.8
P_{O_2} (Torr)	27.4	30.8
pH	7.40	7.38

[a] Mean results of six experiments.
[b] From Battaglia et al. (7).

small if every stream is unsaturated. As a consequence of this fact, a shift to the left of the fetal oxyhemoglobin dissociation curve results both in an increase in saturation and a decrease of umbilical blood P_{O_2}, whereas a shift to the right has the opposite effect (30). This leads to the paradoxical situation that the high oxygen affinity of fetal red cells, whose function is to provide the fetus with adequate oxygen, is also one of the factors that contribute to the low P_{O_2} of fetal blood. The quantitative importance of this contribution, however, is relatively small. Fetal lambs were exchange transfused with adult blood to produce a large right shift of the oxyhemoglobin dissociation curve (7). As shown in Table 6-3, the transfusion caused a marked decrease of umbilical venous oxygen saturation from 79.1 to 51.3% and only a small increase of umbilical venous P_{O_2} from 27.4 to 30.8 Torr. Figure 6-8 illustrates the changes in oxygen saturation and P_{O_2} of fetal blood brought about by a change in the oxyhemoglobin dissociation curve.

To compensate for the relatively low P_{O_2} and oxygen content of fetal blood, the tissues of the fetal lamb are perfused at a high rate. A comparison of the perfusion rates of adult and fetal brain (20) and adult and fetal hind limbs (43) has shown that these regions receive approximately 2.5 times more blood per milliliter of oxygen consumed in the fetus than in the adult. In relation to oxygen demands, the biventricular output of the ovine fetus is almost twice as high as in a mammal at sea level oxygenated by the ventilatory function of the lungs (Chapter 7).

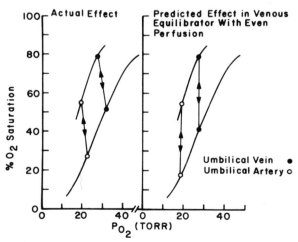

Figure 6-8: Changes in the oxygen affinity of fetal blood have opposite effects on its oxygen saturation and P_{O_2}.

It is apparent that high oxygen affinity and high cardiac output are two complementary aspects of oxygen transport from placenta to fetal tissues. The high oxygen affinity ensures adequate oxygen transfer from placenta to fetal blood, and the high rate of tissue perfusion ensures adequate oxygen transfer from fetal blood to fetal tissues.

As with other mechanisms of physiologic adaptation, both high oxygen affinity and high cardiac output could not be successful if they exceeded certain limits. This is fairly obvious for cardiac output. However, in the case of high oxygen affinity, there seems to be some confusion. For example, Forster (16) questioned the assumption that the high oxygen affinity of fetal red cells is an advantage to the fetus by using a numerical example of fetal oxygen transport in which oxygen affinity of fetal blood was much higher than the actual, normal value for ovine and human fetal blood. He then argued that the high oxygen affinity of fetal blood creates an unnecessarily low tissue P_{O_2} and impedes the transfer of oxygen from blood to tissues. The important issue, however, is whether the actual fetal red cell oxygen affinity is adapted to the actual conditions of fetal oxygenation. To understand the adaptive value of oxygen affinity in any organism, be it prenatal or postnatal, it is essential to keep in mind that hemoglobin must accomplish the dual function of taking up oxygen from the respiratory organ and of unloading oxygen at the tissue level. The experimental data on fetal exchange transfusions (Table 6-3, Figure 6-8) show quite clearly that a decrease in oxygen affinity below its normal value is detrimental to the function of placental uptake of oxygen while simultaneously increasing the P_{O_2} of fetal arterial blood. Itskovitz et al. (17) carried out similar studies in chronically catheterized pregnant sheep and found the same changes in P_{O_2} and oxygen contents in the umbilical venous blood observed in our earlier studies. They found that a fall in umbilical blood flow and in fetal oxygen consumption accompanied the exchange transfusions, confirming that when a low fetal oxygen affinity is coupled with another negative factor impacting on fetal oxygenation, such as a reduction in umbilical blood flow, fetal oxygen consumption is affected.

An increase in oxygen affinity would have the opposite effect, that is, it would improve the oxygen saturation of umbilical venous blood at the cost of reducing arterial and tissue capillary P_{O_2}. Large changes in oxygen affinity in either direction would be lethal. Therefore, in the course of mammalian evolution there must have been selective pressures favoring the production of red cells with an oxygen affinity sufficiently high to attain 80–90% oxygen saturation in umbilical venous blood, yet not so high as to impede the release of oxygen to fetal tissues. The concept that the oxygen affinity of fetal red cells reflects the conditions of maternal-fetal oxygen transfer has important implications in comparative physiology. As we shall see later in this chapter, some species have fetal blood with lower oxygen affinity than ovine and human fetal blood. It follows that the conditions of fetal oxygenation are different in these species.

FETAL CIRCULATORY RESPONSE TO RESPIRATORY GASES

The distribution of oxygen to fetal tissues is controlled by mechanisms that continuously adjust the distribution of fetal cardiac output in response to changes in the level of oxygenation (Chapter 7). Although these adjustments also result in some changes of cardiac output, the salient characteristic of the response is a redistribution of cardiac output. The rate of perfusion of neural and cardiac tissues increases inversely to arterial oxygen content. The blood flows to kidneys, gut, and the nonvisceral parts of the fetus (skeletal muscle, skin, and bones) have a tendency either to increase or to remain constant as the state of fetal oxygenation deteriorates and then to decrease in severe acute hypoxia. Blood flow to the fetal lungs varies directly as a function of pulmonary arterial P_{O_2}. The end result of these multiple and diverse adjustments is that in the fetal lamb, the fraction of cardiac output directed to the central nervous system and heart can vary from approximately 7% in normoxia to as much as 25% in severe hypoxia (41).

EFFECT OF INCREASING MATERNAL P_{O_2} OF INSPIRED AIR ON
FETAL OXYGENATION

Given the many factors that contribute to the production and maintenance of a certain state of fetal oxygenation, there are many ways by which an experimenter can alter this state. The effect of increasing P_{O_2} of inspired air in the mother has received considerable attention because of its potential clinical value. Early studies were inconclusive, probably because they were on acute animal preparations that rapidly deteriorated during the course of the experiment. Some investigators were unable to demonstrate any effect of oxygen administration on fetal oxygenation, some could demonstrate a small increase of fetal arterial P_{O_2} that seemed of negligible value, and some studies even managed to demonstrate an apparent decrease of fetal P_{O_2} and oxygen uptake.

As indicated by the venous equilibration model of the sheep placenta, to understand the effects of elevating P_{O_2} of inspired air it is necessary to focus attention on the relationship between uterine and umbilical venous P_{O_2}. Experiments in chronic sheep preparations have demonstrated conclusively that an increase of uterine venous P_{O_2}, produced either by increasing P_{O_2} of inspired air or by shifting the maternal oxyhemoglobin dissociation curve to the right, is accompanied by a similar increase of umbilical venous P_{O_2} (Figure 6-3). The venous equilibration concept, taken together with the knowledge that variations in maternal arterial P_{O_2} do not appreciably alter uterine and umbilical blood flow (Chapters 7 and 8), can be used to define precisely the effect of maternal hyperoxia on fetal oxygenation. Consider the numerical example in Figure 6-9 which shows blood oxygen content plotted against P_{O_2} for both maternal and fetal blood in sheep. Values for maternal arterial, uterine venous, umbilical venous, and umbilical arterial blood are shown on the curves. Administration of oxygen to the mother causes a large increase of maternal arterial P_{O_2} (step a) and a relatively modest increase (1.0 mM) in arterial oxygen content (step b). If we assume no change in uterine blood flow and oxygen consumption by the uteroplacenta and fetus, the Fick principle demands that uterine venous oxygen content be raised by the same amount (1.0 mM) as arterial oxygen content (step c). If there were an increase in oxygen consumption (as might occur if the fetus had been anoxic prior to oxygen administration) the increase in uterine venous oxygen content would be less. The increase in uterine venous oxygen content causes an increase in uterine venous P_{O_2} (step d). Note that uterine venous P_{O_2} increases much less than maternal arterial P_{O_2} (11.5 versus 410 Torr) because the change in oxygen content takes place on different

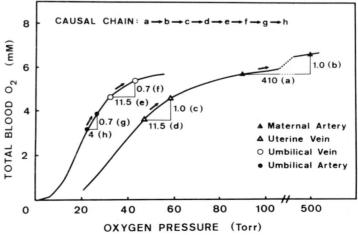

Figure 6-9: Numerical example of the effect of increasing maternal P_{O_2} of inspired air on fetal oxygenation (27).

parts of the oxyhemoglobin dissociation curve. The increase of uterine venous P_{O_2} (11.5 Torr) is followed by an identical increase of umbilical venous P_{O_2} (step e). Note that the oxygen content change is identical in maternal artery and vein, whereas the oxygen tension change is identical in the two venous streams, uterine and umbilical. In any given experimental situation, the changes in umbilical and uterine venous P_{O_2} need not be identical; however, they tend to be similar. The increase in umbilical venous P_{O_2} causes an increase of umbilical venous oxygen content. The magnitude of this increase depends upon the fetal oxyhemoglobin dissociation curve and the fetal oxygen capacity (step f). The increase in umbilical venous oxygen content (0.7 mM) causes the umbilical arterial oxygen content to increase by an approximately equal amount (step g), again as a consequence of the Fick principle. The increase of umbilical arterial oxygen content causes an increase of umbilical arterial P_{O_2} of 4 Torr (step h).

Edelstone *et al.* (14) repeated our earlier studies of the effect of oxygen administration to pregnant ewes upon fetal oxygenation except that the studies were carried out under conditions of a reduction in umbilical blood flow. Under such conditions they were able to demonstrate an increase in fetal oxygen consumption as well as in the level of fetal oxygenation during maternal oxygen administration.

There are two important aspects of the sequence of events shown in Figure 6-9 that deserve emphasis. The first is that the increase in fetal arterial P_{O_2} may be 100-fold less than in the maternal artery (4 versus 410 Torr). This explains why some investigators were unable to detect an increase in fetal P_{O_2}, especially if other important factors that affect fetal oxygenation (e.g., maternal and fetal perfusion of the placenta) were changing at the same time. The second aspect is that the changes in blood oxygen content of maternal and fetal blood are of comparable magnitude (e.g., in Figure 6-9, 1.0 versus 0.7 mM). Indeed, under certain conditions the increase in oxygen content of fetal blood could exceed the maternal. Since the therapeutic aim of oxygen administration is to increase the oxygen content of fetal blood, it would be incorrect to deduce from the relatively small changes of P_{O_2} in fetal blood that an increase of maternal P_{O_2} of inspired air has a negligible effect on fetal oxygenation.

EFFECT OF DECREASING UTERINE BLOOD FLOW
ON FETAL OXYGENATION

According to the Fick principle a decrease of uterine blood flow at constant maternal oxygen capacity and arterial oxygen saturation is bound to produce either a decrease of uterine venous oxygen saturation or a decrease in the oxygen consumption rate of the gravid uterus or both. What actually happens is shown schematically in Figure 6-10, which is based on the results of experiments in sheep in which uterine flow was reduced and kept at a low level for about 1 hr by partial occlusion of the internal common iliac (45). A decrease of uterine blood flow to approximately half the normal level has no effect on oxygen uptake. Therefore, the uterine venous oxygen saturation decreases along the curve predicted by the Fick principle for an organ in which oxygen uptake remains constant. In the example of Figure 6-10, at constant uterine oxygen uptake, the percentage venous oxygen saturation ($\%S_V$) was related to uterine

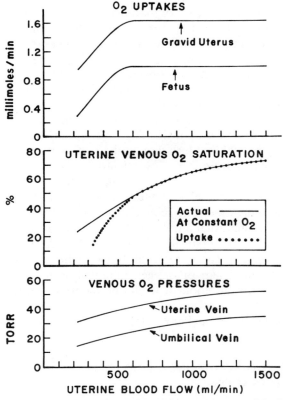

Figure 6-10:   Effect of decreasing uterine blood flow on uterine and fetal oxygen uptakes, uterine venous oxygen saturation, and the P_{O_2} values in uterine venous and umbilical venous blood in a ewe carrying a 3-kg fetus. The figure was constructed using experimental data by Wilkening and Meschia (29, 45).

blood flow (F) (in liters per minute) by the equation

$$\%S_V = 90\left(1 - \frac{1.64}{5.76F}\right) \qquad (6\text{-}3)$$

where 90 is the maternal arterial oxygen saturation percentage, 1.64 is the rate of oxygen consumption by the gravid uterus (in millimoles per minute) and 5.76 is the maternal arterial oxygen content (in millimolar).

As the uterine blood flow decreases further, a point is reached at which the rate of perfusion of the pregnant uterus is no longer sufficient to sustain a normal fetal oxygen uptake. Beyond this point uterine venous oxygen saturation continues to decrease but less than predicted for a constant uterine oxygen uptake.

The decline in uterine venous oxygen saturation is accompanied by a decrease in uterine venous P_{O_2} dictated by the oxyhemoglobin dissociation curve of maternal blood. Note that as uterine blood flow decreases, there is an acidification of uterine venous blood due to a concomitant increase in uterine venous P_{CO_2} (see Figure 6-16). This acidification shifts the maternal oxyhemoglobin dissociation curve to the right (Bohr effect), buffering the decline in P_{O_2}. Nevertheless, the important characteristic is that uterine venous P_{O_2} decreases curvilinearly as a function of uterine blood flow, in the manner indicated in Figure 6-10. The decline in uterine venous P_{O_2} is accompanied by a decline in umbilical venous P_{O_2}. These experimental observations are in agreement with the venous equilibration hypothesis. Of interest is the fact that the uterine venous minus umbilical venous P_{O_2} difference does not decrease at low uterine blood flows. In other words, there is no evidence for any special adaptive mechanism that would make the placental oxygen exchange of respiratory gases more efficient when uterine blood flow is reduced acutely. The effect of uterine blood flow on umbilical venous P_{O_2} may seem small. In our example, a reduction of blood flow from 1500 to 500 ml/min causes a P_{O_2} change of 13 Torr. Nevertheless, the effect of this 13-Torr change on the oxygen saturation and content of fetal blood is profound. As demonstrated in Figure 6-11, fetal arterial oxygen saturation and content decrease to one-third of normal (saturation from 60 to 20% and oxygen content from 4 to 1.3 mM). This is another demonstration of the physiologic importance of small changes of fetal P_{O_2}, reflecting the high oxygen affinity of fetal blood. It is noteworthy that no large increase in umbilical blood flow has been observed in response to an acute decrease in oxygenation of this magnitude. A further reduction of uterine blood flow below the critical level at which the fetus can maintain a normal rate of oxygen consumption causes dramatic changes. The fetus develops a metabolic acidosis which decreases the oxygen affinity of fetal hemoglobin (Bohr effect) and causes a further

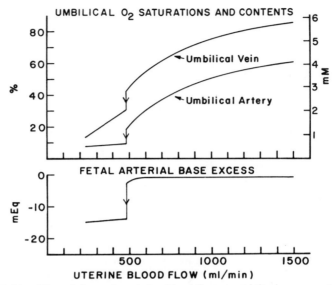

Figure 6-11: Effect of decreasing uterine blood flow on umbilical oxygen saturations and contents and the base excess of fetal blood in a 3-kg sheep fetus. The figure was constructed from experimental data by Wilkening and Meschia (29,45).

reduction in the oxygen saturation of fetal blood. Under these conditions the physiologic state of the fetus is quite unstable and "time dependent." One should regard the values of oxygen consumption and base excess shown in Figures 6-10 and 6-11 for uterine blood flow below 500 ml/min as only indicative of trends within this metastable region of biology. In severe hypoxia, there cannot be any precise relationship between the physiologic state of the fetus and uterine blood flow.

FETAL HYPOXIA

At the outset of a discussion of fetal hypoxia, it is important to note that the word *hypoxia* is a general term used to define a variety of observations in which the level of oxygenation is below standard or control levels. Although such a practice encompasses within this single definition pathologic conditions which are radically different from each other, there are many reports in the literature which treat fetal hypoxia as if it were a single physiologic entity. Frequently, the mean P_{O_2} in one fetal artery has been used as the only index of the hypoxic condition, apparently because the inadequacy of the information provided by such an index is not generally recognized. For example, if one describes fetal hypoxia as a mean arterial P_{O_2} of 13 ± 2 Torr, one is grouping together physiologic states in which arterial oxygen content may range from a level that is still compatible with fetal survival to a level that is an immediate threat to fetal life. This lack of precision in defining fetal hypoxia within studies is further aggravated by the existence of systematic methodologic differences among laboratories. For example, differences in the technique of sampling and in standardization of the electrode may create discrepancies among laboratories of 2–3 Torr for P_{O_2} within the fetal range (i.e., 10–30 Torr range.)

With reference to postnatal life, the fetus is hypoxic. The normal P_{O_2} of fetal arterial blood would be considered excessively low even in mammals living at high altitude. Therefore, it is appropriate to say that the fetus lives in a state of "physiologic hypoxia." This type of hypoxia is physiologic in the sense that it defines a normal state and also because it defines a state in which the rate of oxidative metabolism runs unimpeded by the rate of oxygen supply (Figures 6-10 and 6-11). The use of postnatal life as a standard of reference to define the state of fetal oxygenation as "hypoxic" may seem artificial. However, the concept that the fetus is in a state of physiologic hypoxia helps in our understanding of fetal circulatory physiology as well as the dramatic circulatory changes that take place at birth. Patency of the ductus arteriosus and the high resistance of the fetal pulmonary vascular bed are a result, in part, of the low P_{O_2} of fetal blood (3). The rapid and marked increase of P_{O_2} associated with the onset of breathing is one of the important signals that triggers the circulatory changes of birth. Therefore, an arterial P_{O_2} which is extremely low by postnatal standards is not just a condition that the fetus can tolerate, but a regulator of the fetal circulation. As we have seen, the high rate of fetal cardiac output is also related to the physiologic hypoxia of the fetus.

Stages of Fetal Hypoxia

Starting from a normal level of fetal oxygenation (I, Table 6-4) there are three major stages of acute hypoxia (II–IV, Table 6-4) that one encounters as the oxygen content of fetal blood is decreased by progressively decreasing fetal P_{O_2}. Fetal arterial oxygen content may decrease from its normal level (3–4 mM) to as low as 2.0 mM in the ascending aorta (1.5 mM in the abdominal aorta), with no signs of metabolic acidosis or reduced oxygen uptake (Figure 6-11). This degree of hypoxia (II, Table 6-4) is not an immediate threat to fetal life. However, the margin of safety has decreased to a minimum and the fraction of cardiac output distributed to the heart and central nervous system is approximately twice the normal

Table 6-4

Classification of Hypoxic States in the Fetal Lamb[a]

Type of hypoxia	Approximate range of O_2 in ascending aorta (mM)
I. Physiologic hypoxia	3–4
II. O_2 supply to some tissues is below normal but adequate; absence of metabolic acidosis	2–3
III. O_2 supply is adequate to heart and central nervous system but inadequate to carcass and some viscera; metabolic acidosis	1–2
IV. O_2 supply is inadequate to most of the organism, including central nervous system	<1

[a] From Peeters *et al.* (37).

value (41). Further reduction of arterial oxygen content in the ascending aorta to as low as 1 mM (0.7 mM in the abdominal aorta) creates a situation in which the ability of heart and brain to utilize a normal amount of oxygen is preserved only by diverting to these regions as much as 25% of cardiac output and by depriving less privileged tissues (such as skeletal muscle) of an adequate oxygen supply (37, 41). This degree of hypoxia (III, Table 6-4) is associated with a metabolic acidosis. The final stage (IV, Table 6-4) is reached when the arterial oxygen content in the ascending aorta decreases to such a low level (less than 1.0 mM) that an adequate oxygen supply to heart and brain can no longer be maintained.

In the stage of hypoxia that is compatible with fetal survival and a normal rate of fetal oxygen consumption (II, Table 6-4) the diversion of cardiac output to heart and brain is accomplished by vasodilatation within myocardial and neural tissues without appreciable changes in heart rate and blood pressure. By contrast, rapidly induced severe hypoxia (III and IV, Table 6-4) evokes an increase of blood pressure and bradycardia. The increase in blood pressure is mediated by an outpouring of epinephrine, norepinephrine, and vasopressin which promotes marked vasoconstriction in virtually every major organ (with the exception of the placenta, heart, and brain) assisting in the redistribution of cardiac output and the attainment of maximum perfusion of the heart and central nervous system (Chapter 7).

Fetal bradycardia following each wave of uterine contraction (so-called late deceleration) is used clinically as a sign of fetal hypoxia which is secondary to a reduction of uterine blood flow (Figure 6-12). In sheep, late decelerations that mimic the late decelerations of the human fetus have

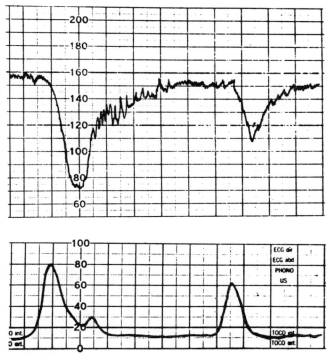

Figure 6-12:   Example of fetal bradycardia (top panel) following each wave of uterine contractions (lower panel). Heart rate is in beats per minute, amniotic pressure is in Torr (11).

been produced by short, periodic occlusions of the maternal common internal iliac artery feeding the uterine arteries (36). Barcroft first demonstrated that the response of the mature ovine fetal heart to acute, severe hypoxia is a vagal reflex that can be abolished by atropine (4). Even in the absence of vagal stimulation, however, asphyxia will eventually produce a fetal bradycardia via a direct effect of oxygen deprivation on cardiac function. In a fetus that is already in stage II or III of hypoxia, the superposition of uterine contractions could produce a slowing of the heart which could be misinterpreted as reflex bradycardia, but is in fact the sign of inadequate oxygen supply to the heart (36).

Chronic fetal hypoxia, i.e., a persistent level of oxygenation which is less than optimal, is a rather common occurrence. Early investigations of fetal life were based on the expectation that fetal blood pH and oxygen saturation would be well regulated and exhibit a narrow range of interani-

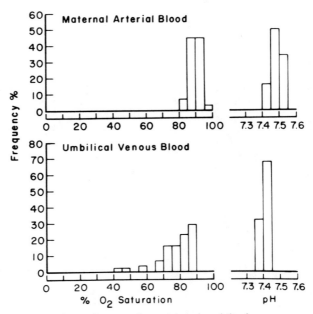

Figure 6-13: Comparison of maternal arterial and umbilical venous oxygen saturation and pH.

mal variability. Figure 6-13 shows that in unstressed ewes the range of variation of fetal blood pH is indeed narrow, but the range of variation of oxygen saturation is much wider in umbilical venous blood, the most oxygenated fetal blood, than in maternal arterial blood. In Figure 6-13 almost half of the 56 animals studied over a 17-month period had umbilical venous oxygen saturations below 80%. Unfortunately, we know very little about the causative factors of this variability. The specific aspects of placental respiratory function which vary markedly among pregnant animals of the same species are not yet known nor do we know the hormonal or other factors which regulate the growth of the placenta and its vasculature and thus determine whether the placenta of one animal is a better respiratory organ than the placenta of another animal. It is interesting to note that among the fetuses presented in Figure 6-13, those with umbilical venous oxygen saturations below 50% had placentas that weighed approximately one-third of normal but were otherwise of normal appearance. These observations provide an experimental basis for the concept that various degrees of "placental insufficiency" do exist even in the absence of obvious placental pathology.

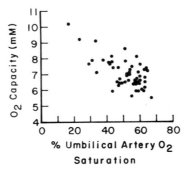

Figure 6-14: Relationship of fetal blood oxygen capacity to arterial oxygen saturation in chronic fetal sheep preparations.

REGULATION OF FETAL BLOOD OXYGEN CAPACITY

In well oxygenated fetal lambs (umbilical venous oxygen saturation >80%), oxygen capacity is approximately 6.7 mM (6.7 $\pm$ 0.64 SD) and slightly higher on the average than maternal oxygen capacity (6.3 $\pm$ 0.49 SD). Given the extremely low P_{O_2} of fetal blood, the existence of only a small discrepancy between maternal and fetal hemoglobin levels may suggest the absence of a regulatory influence of oxygen on fetal hemoglobin synthesis. This is not the case, however. Fetal erythropoietin levels increase sharply when fetal blood volume is reduced by bleeding (48). Injection of antierythropoietin serum in fetal sheep produces a decrease of circulating reticulocytes and a reduced rate of radioactive iron incorporation into spleen and bone marrow (47). Furthermore, chronic suboptimal levels of fetal oxygen saturation tend to be associated with high levels of fetal hemoglobin (Figure 6-14). Taken together, these bits of information indicate that the rate of fetal hemoglobin synthesis is regulated by the P_{O_2} of fetal blood, but with a different "setting" so that the fetal organism does not react to its physiologic hypoxia by producing abnormally large quantities of hemoglobin. The fact that the production of erythropoietin in the fetus is not localized in the kidneys (48) as in adult mammals but in the liver (38) is perhaps related to this adaptation of the fetal erythropoietic system to the fetal environment.

COMPARATIVE ASPECTS OF FETAL RESPIRATORY PHYSIOLOGY

The sheep placenta is the prototype of an exchanger with a low degree of effectiveness. Placental effectiveness in other mammals is higher than in sheep and may come fairly close to the maximal, ideal effectiveness of a countercurrent exchanger (Chapter 2). The best evidence for the existence of placental types with a high degree of effectiveness is in guinea pigs, but there is histologic and/or functional evidence showing that countercurrent-like systems of placental exchange are present in mammals as diverse as small rodents, rabbits, and the horse (Chapter 1 and 2). The investigation of placental respiratory function in these mammals has shown a remarkable interspecies difference in the way in which a high degree of placental effectiveness is put to use.

In guinea pigs and rabbits the maternal placental blood flow of late gestation, expressed either per gram of fetus or per rate of oxygen uptake by the conceptus, is approximately one-half to one-third the comparable value in sheep (Chapter 8). As a consequence, despite the more efficient placenta, the guinea pig and rabbit fetuses have a degree of physiologic hypoxia similar to that observed in the ovine fetus. Although measurements of fetal P_{O_2} in small mammals must be interpreted with caution, there is good evidence that the blood of fetal guinea pigs and rabbits near term has a high oxygen affinity (32). In rabbits, the P_{50} of fetal red cells declines from 29 to 20 Torr in the last half of gestation (19). The decline is due primarily to a decrease of acid-soluble phosphate compounds in the red cells and is concomitant with a decline in uterine venous P_{O_2}. The conclusion from this evidence is that guinea pig and rabbits are examples of mammals in which a high degree of placental effectiveness translates into a low level of maternal placental perfusion and into a fetal environment similar, in late gestation, to the fetal environment of mammals with less effective placentas. In Chapter 2, we referred to this type of placenta as a "countercurrent exchanger with maternal advantage."

In the horse, a species in which there is structural evidence of a countercurrent arrangement of maternal and fetal placental vessels, fetal umbilical venous P_{O_2} is much higher than in sheep (48.4 ± 0.7 Torr) and the oxygen affinity of fetal blood is relatively low (12). In four fetuses, the P_{50} at pH 7.4 and 39°C ranged between 27.9 and 31.9 Torr. Furthermore, uterine blood flow expressed per rate of oxygen uptake by the pregnant uterus or per kilogram of tissue is as high as in sheep (42). Thus, it would appear that in the horse the high effectiveness of the placenta translates into a relatively high level of umbilical venous P_{O_2} and no decrease in maternal placental blood flow. The placenta of the domestic cat may be another example of an exchanger in which a high level of effectiveness is used to equilibrate umbilical venous blood with a high P_{O_2} rather than to decrease the level of maternal placental perfusion. This supposition is based on the single bit of evidence that the oxygen affinity of fetal blood is relatively low in the cat (P_{50} = 35.6 ± 0.9 Torr at pH 7.4 and 38°C) and equal to the affinity of maternal blood (34). Furthermore, no fetal hemoglobin has been detected in the cat (34). The horse and cat placentas may be examples of countercurrent exchangers with fetal advantage (Chapter 2).

The effectiveness of the human placenta has been a matter of speculation. It is not unusual to find in the literature the claim that the human placenta is a countercurrent exchange system (46) despite the fact that there is no evidence for such a claim. On the basis of histologic observations, the human placenta has been described as a multicapillary system (Figure 2-2, Chapter 2) which is a system with a fairly high flow-limited effectiveness (5). However, data on oxygen transfer make us question whether the level of performance of the human placenta as an organ of diffusional exchange is any higher than that of the ovine placenta. In the rhesus monkey, an animal with a placental histology similar to that in humans, uterine and umbilical venous P_{O_2} values were measured before and during administration of oxygen to the mother. The umbilical venous P_{O_2} rose only from 22 to 30 mmHg with oxygen breathing and remained 15 mmHg lower than the uterine venous P_{O_2} (8). Wulf *et al.* (46) measured the P_{O_2} of umbilical venous and maternal arterial blood while pregnant patients were breathing different gas mixtures. By changing the maternal arterial P_{O_2} from 38 to 583 mmHg, they obtained a much smaller increment of umbilical venous P_{O_2}, from 17.8 to 39.8 mmHg. These results are indistinguishable from results obtained in studying the respiratory function of the ovine placenta and can be readily explained if we assume that the venous equilibration model is applicable to the human placenta. Table 6-5 provides a summary of the species differences we have discussed.

Table 6-5

Interspecies Differences in Placental Respiratory Function

Placental type	Species[a]
I. Venous equilibration exchanger with high level of maternal perfusion and fetal blood with low P_{O_2} and high O_2 affinity	Sheep, goat (cattle, pig, rhesus monkey, humans)
II. Countercurrent exchanger with low level of maternal perfusion and fetal blood with low P_{O_2} and high O_2 affinity	Guinea pig, rabbit (small rodents)
III. Countercurrent exchanger with high level of maternal perfusion and fetal blood with relatively high P_{O_2} and low O_2 affinity	(Horse, cat)

[a] Included in parentheses are species for which the placement is tentative.

FETAL ACID–BASE BALANCE

On a molar basis, fetal CO_2 production rate is approximately equal to fetal oxygen consumption rate (18). The CO_2 produced by the fetal tissues is carried via the umbilical circulation to the placenta, where it diffuses into the maternal blood that perfuses the pregnant uterus. The CO_2 excretion from the fetus across the placenta represents the largest irreversible loss of carbon from the fetal compartment. Note that fetal CO_2 excretion is not the only contribution to the uptake of CO_2 by the uterine circulation. There is an additional rate of CO_2 uptake representing the CO_2 production of the placenta and uterus.

Early studies carried out acutely in pregnant rabbits (10) demonstrated the fact that P_{CO_2} equilibrates rapidly across the rabbit placenta (Figure 6-15). The diffusion of CO_2 from fetus to mother requires the maintenance of a P_{CO_2} gradient between fetal and maternal blood. The magnitude of this gradient depends upon the effectiveness of the placental exchange process. In sheep the uterine and umbilical circulations form a "venous equilibrator," that is, an exchange system that tends to equilibrate the uterine and umbilical venous concentrations of highly diffusible mole-

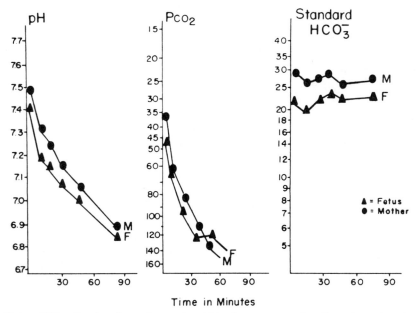

Figure 6-15:   Results of experiments in rabbits demonstrating the effect of CO_2 breathing (8% CO_2 in inspired air) on maternal and fetal blood pH, P_{CO_2}, and standard bicarbonate (10).

cules (Chapter 2). In agreement with this knowledge, the umbilical venous P_{CO_2} of sheep fetuses has been shown to be somewhat higher than, and to vary as a function of, uterine venous P_{CO_2}. The most convincing evidence comes from observations describing the effect of decreasing uterine blood flow on the P_{CO_2} of maternal and fetal blood (45). Under normal physiologic conditions, the P_{CO_2} of uterine venous blood is 2–4 Torr higher than the P_{CO_2} of maternal arterial blood. When uterine blood flow is decreased experimentally by means of an occluder around the terminal aorta, the P_{CO_2} difference between uterine venous and arterial blood widens to as much as 15 Torr (Figure 6-16) because the CO_2 entering the uterine circulation from the placenta is taken up by a smaller quantity of maternal blood. As uterine venous P_{CO_2} increases in response to a decrease in the rate of uterine perfusion, umbilical venous P_{CO_2} increases in close relation to uterine venous P_{CO_2} (Figure 6-17). Under normal physiologic conditions the umbilical venous P_{CO_2} of sheep is approximately 3 Torr higher than uterine venous P_{CO_2}. There are several possible reasons for this difference. The release of CO_2 from fetal blood and its uptake by maternal blood may be too slow for complete equilibration of the two blood streams. In addition, placental CO_2 production and the ineffectiveness of the placental exchanger must contribute to the maintenance of an umbili-

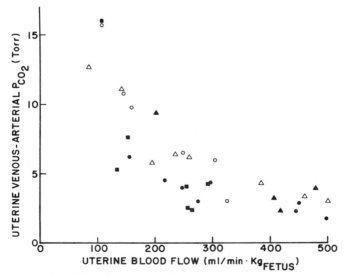

Figure 6-16:   Effect of decreasing uterine blood flow on the uterine venous–arterial difference of P_{CO_2}. Each animal is represented by a separate symbol. The figure was constructed from experimental data by Wilkening and Meschia (45).

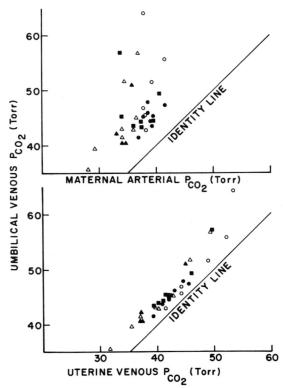

Figure 6-17:   In sheep, umbilical venous P_{CO_2} is more closely related to uterine venous P_{CO_2} than to maternal arterial P_{CO_2}. Each animal is represented by a separate symbol (45).

cal–uterine venous P_{CO_2} difference. However, the relative importance of each of these factors has not been analyzed.

Under pathologic conditions, fetal P_{CO_2} can be either below (respiratory alkalosis) or above (respiratory acidosis) normal. Fetal respiratory alkalosis is a consequence of maternal hyperventilation, which decreases maternal arterial P_{CO_2} and in turn decreases uterine venous P_{CO_2} and the P_{CO_2} of fetal blood. A high placental blood flow cannot contribute significantly to fetal respiratory alkalosis because the venous–arterial P_{CO_2} difference across the pregnant uterus is already small (2–4 Torr) under normal physiologic conditions. By contrast, fetal respiratory acidosis can result from maternal hypoventilation or impaired placental CO_2 transfer or both. Maternal hypoventilation causes an increase of maternal arterial P_{CO_2}, which in turn increases the P_{CO_2} with which fetal blood equilibrates. At normal levels of maternal arterial P_{CO_2}, fetal arterial P_{CO_2} can be elevated above normal as a consequence of underperfusion of the placenta by the mother and/or fetus.

Normally, in chronic sheep preparations the pH of fetal arterial blood varies within the range of 7.32 to 7.42. In considering the factors that regulate fetal pH, it is important to focus attention on the permeability characteristics of the placental barrier. If the placenta were a metabolically inert, semipermeable membrane that permitted the rapid equilibration of ions, fetal plasma pH would tend to bear a constant relationship to maternal plasma pH and could not be regulated independently. In sheep, however, the transfer of ions across the placenta is very slow. Thus, if a transplacental gradient of hydrogen ions is established by the infusion of NH_4Cl into either the mother or the fetus, it persists for several hours. During starvation, the metabolic acidosis due to accumulation of ketoacids is limited to the maternal compartment and fetal arterial pH can become equal to or exceed maternal arterial pH (Figure 6-18). From such

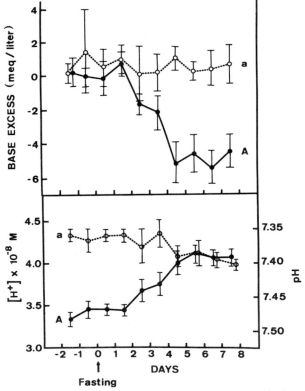

Figure 6-18:   Ovine fetal (a) and maternal (A) arterial base excess and hydrogen ion activity ($\pm$ SEM) before and during fasting (40).

evidence it would seem that the ovine fetus has autonomous control of its bicarbonate concentration, presumably via regulation of fetal renal function. There are no studies of acid base regulation in the nephrectomized fetal lamb, and no attempts have been made to establish the relative contribution of the placenta, the fetal kidneys, and other organs (for example, the fetal lungs) in the chronic regulation of fetal bicarbonate concentration.

These results in sheep demonstrating that the bicarbonate concentrations of maternal and fetal extracellular fluids can vary independently cannot be generalized to other species. There are substantial differences among mammals in the permeability of the placental barrier to ions. The hemochorial placenta of the rhesus monkey has been shown to be much more permeable to chloride ions than the epitheliochorial placentas of sheep and goats (6). In these species, and perhaps in humans, metabolic disturbances of acid-base balance in the mother would probably cause analogous disturbances in the fetus. However, there is no exact information in humans or any other species with a hemochorial placenta about the rate at which a metabolic disturbance of acid-base balance in the maternal compartment is transmitted to the fetal compartment. Note that even in primates, ions such as Na and Cl have much lower placental clearances than highly diffusible molecules such as antipyrine and tritiated water (6).

FETAL LUNGS

The fetal lungs secrete fluid that flows out of the trachea to be swallowed and/or excreted into the amnion. In the last month of gestation the lungs of fetal sheep secrete fluid at the rate of approximately 4 ml/kg/hr (26). Approximately 2 days before birth, lung fluid production decreases (21). In comparison to fetal plasma, fetal lung fluid has a high concentration of chloride ions (157 versus 107 mEq) and a low concentration of bicarbonate ions and proteins (Chapter 9). According to Olver and Strang (35), a chloride ion pump is responsible for the active transfer of chloride ions from fetal blood into pulmonary fluid.

During fetal apnea, the lung fluid is under a positive pressure of about 1.5–3 Torr with respect to the amnion (23). Periodically, the fetus makes rapid, irregular breathing movements that occur up to 40% of the time (13). These movements produce a small tidal volume of less than 1 ml but create a negative tracheal pressure of 5 to 10 Torr. In addition, there are occasional more vigorous movements ("gasps") that produce greater pressure changes. Fetal breathing activity generally coincides with low voltage electrocortical activity (REM sleep) (13). The incidence of breathing movements and the magnitude of the pressure changes can be increased by fetal hypercapnia (9), the induction of fetal metabolic acidosis (33), or the fetal infusion of prostaglandin synthesis inhibitors (22). One of the functions of fetal breathing is to promote development of the respiratory muscles. Section of the phrenic nerves in fetal lambs leads to atrophy of the diaphragm (2). Both lung fluid production and breathing movements seem to be important in the regulation of lung growth. If the fetal trachea is ligated, the lungs become distended with fluid and pulmonary wet weight even after fluid drainage at autopsy is increased. On the other hand, the continuous collection of tracheal fluid by means of a cannula that connects the fetal trachea with the outside tends to decrease lung size (1). Transection of the spinal cord above the phrenic nucleus abolishes fetal breathing and results in pulmonary hypoplasia (23, 44). These experiments suggest that the intrapulmonary pressure exerted by lung fluid and the periodic oscillations in pulmonary transmural pressure caused by breathing are necessary in stimulating the growth of the fetal lungs.

One of the most important events in fetal lung maturation is the synthesis and secretion of the pulmonary surface active agent (surfactant). At about 60% gestation in human pregnancy, there is a rapid increase in the synthesis, and storage of lecithin, which is a major component of surfactant. A relatively small amount of the lecithin produced within the fetal lungs is secreted into the alveoli and appears in the amniotic fluid. Changes in amniotic fluid phospholipids are used for the clinical assessment of fetal maturity (Chapter 9).

Fetal lung maturation is under hormonal control. This control is complex, both in terms of the different aspects of maturation that can be the target of hormone action (e.g., alveolar structure, surfactant synthesis, and secretion) and in terms of the hormones involved and their interrelationships. In the ovine fetus, lung maturation is associated with the rapid increase in plasma cortisol concentration that precedes birth. Cortisol infusion in a premature lamb fetus triggers parturition and accelerates lung maturation. However, in the hypophysectomized fetus the infusion of ACTH, but not cortisol, restores lung maturation to normal (23).

REFERENCES

1. Alcorn, D., Adamson, T.M., Lambert, T.F., Maloney, J.E., Ritchie, B.C. and Robinson, P.M. (1977). *Morphological effects of tracheal ligation and drainage in the fetal lamb.* Journal of Anatomy **123,** 649–660.
2. Alcorn, D., Adamson, T.M., Maloney, J.E. and Robinson, P.M. (1980). *Morphological effects of either chronic bilateral phrenectomy or vagotomy in the fetal lamb lung.* Journal of Anatomy **130,** 683–695.

3. Assali, N.S. and Brinkman, C.R. (1972). *Control of systemic and pulmonary vasomotor tone before and after birth.* In "Comparative Pathophysiology of Circulatory Disturbances" (C.M. Bloor, ed.), pp 13–37, Plenum Publishing Co., New York.

4. Barcroft, J. (1947). "Researches on Prenatal Life." Charles C. Thomas Publishers, Springfield, Illinois.

5. Bartels, H. and Moll, W. (1964). *Passage of inert substances and oxygen in the human placenta.* Pfluegers Archives Gesamte Physiologie Menschen Tiere **280,** 165–177.

6. Battaglia, F.C., Behrman, R.E., Meschia, G., Seeds, A.E. and Bruns, P.B. (1968). *Clearance of inert molecules, Na and Cl ions across the primate placenta.* American Journal of Obstetrics and Gynecology **102,** 1135–1143.

7. Battaglia, F.C., Bowes, W., McGaughey, H.R., Makowski, E.L. and Meschia, G. (1969). *The effect of fetal exchange transfusions with adult blood upon fetal oxygenation.* Pediatric Research **3,** 60–65.

8. Behrman, R.E., Peterson, E.N. and Delannoy, C.W. (1969). *The supply of O_2 to the primate fetus with two different O_2 tensions and anesthetics.* Respiratory Physiology **6,** 271–283.

9. Boddy, K., Dawes, G.S., Fisher, R., Pinter, S. and Robinson, J.S. (1974). *Foetal respiratory movements, electrocortical and cardiovascular responses to hypoxaemia and hypercapnia in sheep.* Journal of Physiology **243,** 599–618.

10. Bruns, P.D., Bowes, W.A. Jr., Drose, V.E. and Battaglia, F.C. (1963). *Effect of respiratory acidosis on the rabbit fetus in utero.* American Journal of Obstetrics and Gynecology **87,** 1074–1080.

11. Cibils, L.A. (1981). "Electronic Fetal–Maternal Monitoring. Antepartum, Intrapartum," PSG Publishing, Co., Inc., Boston.

12. Comline, R.S. and Silver, M. (1974). *A comparative study of blood gas tensions, oxygen affinity and red cell 2,3-DPG concentrations in foetal and maternal blood in the mare, cow and sow.* Journal of Physiology (London) **242,** 805–826.

13. Dawes, G.S., Fox, H.E., Leduc, B.M., Liggins, G.C. and Richards, R.T. (1972). *Respiratory movements and rapid eye movement sleep in the foetal lamb.* Journal of Physiology (London) **220,** 119–143.

14. Edelstone, D.I., Peticca, B.B. and Goldblum, L.J. (1985). *Effects of maternal oxygen administration on fetal oxygenation during reductions in umbilical blood flow in fetal lambs.* American Journal of Obstetrics and Gynecology **152,** 351–358.

15. Evans, J.V. and Turner, H.N. (1965). *Haemoglobin type and reproductive performance in Australian Merino sheep.* Nature **207,** 1396–1397.

16. Forster, R.E. II. (1973). *Some principles governing maternal–foetal transfer of the placenta.* In "Proceedings of the Sir Joseph Barcroft Centenary Symposium on Foetal and Neonatal Physiology," pp 223–237, University Press, Cambridge, England.

17. Itskovitz, J., Goetzman, B.W., Roman, C. and Rudolph, A.M. (1984). *Effects of fetal–maternal exchange transfusion on fetal oxygenation and blood flow distribution.* American Journal of Physiology **247,** H655–H660.

18. James, E.J., Raye, J.R., Gresham, E.L., Makowski, E.L., Meschia, G. and Battaglia, F.C. (1972). *Fetal oxygen consumption, carbon dioxide production and glucose uptake in a chronic sheep preparation.* Pediatrics **50,** 361–371.

19. Jelkmann, W. and Bauer, C. (1977). *Oxygen affinity and phosphate compounds of red blood cells during intrauterine development of rabbits.* Pflugers Archives **372,** 149–156.

20. Jones, M.D. Jr., Burd, L.I., Makowski, E.L., Meschia, G. and Battaglia, F.C. (1975). *Cerebral metabolism in sheep: A comparative study of the adult, the lamb and the fetus.* American Journal of Physiology **229,** 235–239.

21. Kitterman, J.A., Ballard, P.L., Clements, J.A., et al. (1979). *Tracheal fluid in fetal lambs: Spontaneous decrease prior to birth.* Journal of Applied Physiology **47**, 985–989.
22. Kitterman, J.A., Liggins, G.C., Clements, J.A. and Tooley, W.H. (1979). *Stimulation of breathing movements in fetal sheep by inhibitors of prostaglandin synthesis.* Journal of Developmental Physiology **1**, 453–466.
23. Liggins, G.C. and Kitterman, J.A. (1981). *Development of the fetal lung.* In "The Fetus and Independent Life," Ciba Foundation Symposium 86, pp 308–322, Pitman Ltd., London.
24. Longo, L.D. and Ching, K.S. (1977). *Placental diffusing capacity for carbon monoxide and oxygen in unanesthetized sheep.* Journal of Applied Physiology **43**, 885–893.
25. Longo, L.D., Power, G.G. and Forster, R.E. II. (1969). *Placental diffusing capacity for carbon monoxide at varying partial pressures of oxygen.* Journal of Applied Physiology **26**, 360–370.
26. Mescher, E.J., Platzker, A.C.G., Ballard, P.L., Kitterman, J.A., Clements, J.A. and Tooley, W.H. (1975). *Ontogeny of tracheal fluids, pulmonary surfactant and plasma corticoids in the fetal lamb.* Journal of Applied Physiology **39**, 1017–1021.
27. Meschia, G. (1977). *Transfer of oxygen across the placenta.* In "Intrauterine Asphyxia and the Developing Fetal Brain" (L. Gluck, ed.), Year Book Medical Publishers, Inc., Chicago.
28. Meschia, G. (1979). *Supply of oxygen to the fetus.* Journal of Reproductive Medicine **23**, 160–165.
29. Meschia, G. (1985). *Safety margin of fetal oxygenation.* Journal of Reproductive Medicine **30**, 308–311.
30. Meschia, G., Battaglia, F.C., Makowski, E.L. and Droegemueller, W. (1969). *Effect of varying umbilical blood O_2 affinity on umbilical vein P_{O_2}.* Journal of Applied Physiology **26**, 410–416.
31. Meschia, G., Battaglia, F.C., Hay, W.W. Jr. and Sparks, J.W. (1980). *Utilization of substrates by the ovine placenta in vivo.* Federation Proceedings **39**, 245–249.
32. Metcalfe, J., Dhindsa, D.S. and Novy, M.J. (1973). *General aspects of oxygen transport in maternal and fetal blood.* In "Proceedings of the Sir Joseph Barcroft Centenary Symposium on Foetal and Neonatal Physiology," pp 63–73, University Press, Cambridge, England.
33. Molteni, R.A., Melmed, M.H., Sheldon, R.E., Jones, M.D. and Meschia, G. (1980). *Induction of fetal breathing by metabolic acidemia and its effect on blood flow to the respiratory muscles.* American Journal of Obstetrics and Gynecology **136**, 609–620.
34. Novy, M.J. and Parer, J.T. (1969). *Absence of high blood oxygen affinity in the fetal cat.* Respiratory Physiology **6**, 144–150.
35. Olver, R.E. and Strang, L.B. (1974). *Ion fluxes across the pulmonary epithelium and the secretion of lung liquid in the foetal lamb.* Journal of Physiology **241**, 327–357.
36. Parer, J.T. (1980). *Fetal O_2 consumption and mechanisms of fetal heart rate response during artificially produced late decelerations of the fetal heart in sheep.* American Journal of Obstetrics and Gynecology **136**, 478–482.
37. Peeters, L.L.H., Sheldon, R.E., Jones, M.D. Jr., Makowski, E.L. and Meschia, G. (1979). *Blood flow to fetal organs as a function of arterial oxygen content.* American Journal of Obstetrics and Gynecology **135**, 637–646.
38. Peschle, C., Marone, G., Genovese, A., Cillo, C., Magli, C. and Condorelli, M. (1976). *Erythropoietin production by the liver in fetal–neonatal life.* Life Sciences **17**, 1325–1330.
39. Rankin, J.H.G., Meschia, G., Makowski, E.L. and Battaglia, F.C. (1971). *Relationship*

between uterine and umbilical venous P_{O_2} *in sheep.* American Journal of Physiology **220**, 1688–1692.

40. Schreiner, R.L., Burd, L.I., Jones, M.D. Jr., Lemons, J.A., Sheldon, R.E., Simmons, M.A., Battaglia, F.C. and Meschia, G. (1978). *Fetal metabolism in fasting sheep. In* "Fetal and Newborn Cardiovascular Physiology," (L.D. Longo and D.D. Reneau, eds.), Volume 2, pp 197–222, Garland STPM Press, New York.

41. Sheldon, R.E., Peeters, L.L.H., Jones, M.D. Jr., Makowski, E.L. and Meschia, G. (1979). *Redistribution of cardiac output and oxygen delivery in the hypoxemic fetal lamb.* American Journal of Obstetrics and Gynecology **135**, 1071–1078.

42. Silver, M. and Comline, R.S. (1975). *Transfer of gases and metabolites in the equine placenta: A comparison with other species.* Journal of Reproduction and Fertility (Supplement) **23**, 589–594.

43. Singh, S., Sparks, J.W., Meschia, G., Battaglia, F.C. and Makowski, E.L. (1984). *Comparison of fetal and maternal hindlimb metabolic quotients in sheep.* American Journal of Obstetrics and Gynecology **149**, 441–449.

44. Wigglesworth, J.S. and Desai, R. (1979). *Effects on lung growth of cervical cord section in the rabbit fetus.* Early Human Development **3**, 51–65.

45. Wilkening, R.B. and Meschia, G. (1983). *Fetal oxygen uptake, oxygenation, and acid-base balance as a function of uterine blood flow.* American Journal of Physiology **244**, H749–H755.

46. Wulf, K.H., Kunzel, W. and Lehmann, V. (1972). *Clinical aspects of placental gas exchange. In* "Respiratory Gas Exchange and Blood Flow in the Placenta" (L.D. Longo and H. Bartels, eds.), DHEW Publication (NIH) #73-361, Washington, D.C.

47. Zanjani, E.D., Mann, L.I., Burlington, H., Gordon, A.S. and Wasserman, L.R. (1974). *Evidence for a physiologic role of erythropoietin in fetal erythropoiesis.* Blood **44**, 285–290.

48. Zanjani, E.D., Peterson, E.N., Gordon, A.S. and Wasserman, L.R. (1974). *Erythropoietin production in the fetus: Role of the kidney and maternal anemia.* Journal of Laboratory and Clinical Medicine **83**, 281–287.

7
Fetal Circulatory Physiology

The circulatory system of the fetus, depicted in Figure 7-1 (5), is radically different from that of postnatal life. Blood carrying oxygen and nutrients flows from the placenta to the fetus via the umbilical vein. Some of the umbilical venous blood bypasses the liver and enters directly into the inferior vena cava (IVC) via the *ductus venosus*. The remainder perfuses the liver. The left hepatic lobe is perfused almost exclusively by umbilical venous blood, whereas the right lobe receives a nearly equal contribution from the portal vein and from the umbilical vein (12). The hepatic artery contributes less than 10% of liver flow in the fetal lamb (12). Within the thoracic IVC, blood from the *ductus venosus*, hepatic veins, and abdominal IVC mix and flow toward the heart to be routed in two different directions: (a) through the *foramen ovale* and left atrium into the left ventricle and (b) through the right atrium into the right ventricle. Normally, venous return via the superior vena cava (SVC) is routed entirely into the right ventricle. The mixing of ductal, hepatic, and abdominal IVC blood in the thoracic IVC is incomplete (13). Blood flowing through the *ductus venosus* and left hepatic lobe streams preferentially toward the *foramen ovale* and the left heart.

Most of the output of the right ventricle bypasses the lungs, which have a high vascular resistance, and flows through the *ductus arteriosus* into the aorta. In the normal fetus the *ductus arteriosus* is a wide open, large vessel that has the same diameter as the main pulmonary artery. Upon entering the aorta, the blood from the *ductus arteriosus* mixes with blood

189

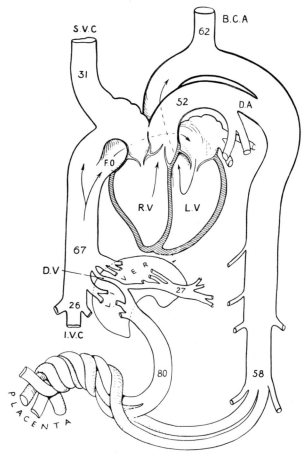

Figure 7-1: Diagram of the fetal circulation. The numbers indicate the percentage of oxygen saturation of blood withdrawn simultaneously from various vessels and averaged from determinations on six fetal lambs. I.V.C., *inferior vena cava;* D.V., *ductus venosus;* S.V.C., *superior vena cava;* F.O., *foramen ovale;* D.A., *ductus arteriosus;* B.C.A., *brachiocephalic artery* (5).

flowing from ascending to descending aorta, through the aortic isthmus, to form the blood that perfuses the lower body and the placenta. The heart and the upper body are perfused exclusively by blood ejected from the left ventricle.

The functional meaning of the *ductus venosus* is uncertain. It represents a low resistance channel for the passage of blood from the umbilical vein to the thoracic IVC, presumably to minimize venous pressure within the umbilical circulation. To the contrary, the main functional meaning of the *foramen ovale* and the *ductus arteriosus* is fairly obvious. The com-

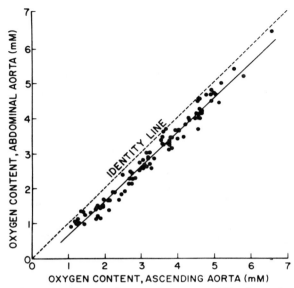

Figure 7-2: Relationship between the oxygen contents of blood samples drawn simultaneously from the abdominal and ascending aorta of fetal lambs and at different levels of maternal oxygenation (40).

bined output of the fetal heart would have to be almost twice its actual value if most of the blood circulating through the fetus and the placenta did not bypass the lungs via the *foramen ovale* and the *ductus arteriosus*. Two shunts (foramen and ductus) are needed to ensure that venous return is apportioned about equally between right and left ventricles.

The routing of SVC flow into the right ventricle and the preferential streaming of *ductus venosus* blood and left hepatic blood into the left ventricle produce a pattern of perfusion in which the fetal upper body is better oxygenated than the lungs and the fetal lower body. In the sheep fetus the oxygen content difference between ascending and abdominal aorta is approximately 0.4 mM, a difference that is fairly constant at oxygen content levels in the descending aorta greater than 1.5 mM (Figure 7-2) (40). Such a difference in oxygen content between the ascending and abdominal aorta may have survival value during hypoxia by contributing to the preferential oxygenation of brain and heart.

CARDIAC OUTPUT

In postnatal life the term *cardiac output* is used to define the output of either the left or right ventricle because the two ventricles work in series and have equal input and output values. In fetal life the right and left ventricles may have different outputs and both pump blood into the systemic circulation. For this reason, the common definition of cardiac output employed in postnatal life is inapplicable to fetal life. In fetal physiology *cardiac output* generally means the combined output of the two ventricles, although there are instances in which the expression *fetal cardiac output* has been used to denote the combined ventricular output minus pulmonary and/or coronary flows. The first measurements of fetal cardiac output in the nonexteriorized fetal lamb were made by Rudolph and Heymann in 1967 (36). These investigators introduced into fetal physiology the microsphere technique, which allows an estimate of blood flow to any organ or regions of the fetus and the placenta. Several versions of this technique have been used since then to satisfy the needs of special experimental situations and to improve the accuracy of the results. Microspheres of 15 or 25 μM diameter are injected into the fetal IVC and are carried to the right and left fetal ventricles. Each ventricle acts as a mixing chamber for the uniform distribution of the particles. The spheres are ejected by the heart and carried to the body tissues where they are trapped in the microcirculation. The amount of microspheres trapped in each organ is proportional to the blood flow to that organ. In order to use this principle to quantify organ blood flows, it is necessary to measure the amount of microspheres trapped in a reference organ whose blood flow is measured by some independent method, or, more conveniently, to measure the amount of microspheres collected in a reference blood sample drawn at a constant and known rate. Therefore, fetal cardiac output and its distribution can be measured by injecting a bolus of radioactively labeled microspheres into the fetal IVC, while simultaneously withdrawing three reference samples: (a) from the fetal abdominal aorta below the confluence of the *ductus arteriosus;* (b) from the brachiocephalic artery; and (c) from the right ventricle or main pulmonary artery. At autopsy the fetus is divided into three parts: lungs, tissues perfused exclusively by blood ejected from the left ventricle (heart and upper body), and tissues perfused by the abdominal aorta (lower body and placenta). The appropriate reference samples are then used to calculate: pulmonary flow, flow to the upper body, and flow to the lower body and placenta. The sum of these three flows is the combined output of the fetal heart, that is, fetal cardiac output.

The cardiac output of the mature fetal lamb *in utero* has been measured by several investigators each using a modification of the basic microsphere method (Table 7-1), with substantial agreement on a value of approximately 500 ml/kg/min.

The microsphere technique has also been used to calculate the relative

Table 7-1

Combined Ventricular Output in
the Mature Fetal Lamb

Reference	n^a	Cardiac output $(ml/kg/min)^b$
37	10	548 ± 20
33	9	463 ± 7
15	10	592 ± 28
2	12	462 ± 56

[a] Number of observations.
[b] Values are expressed as mean ± SEM. Units are milliliters of blood per kilogram of fetal body weight per minute.

contributions of the right and left ventricle to the combined fetal cardiac output and to calculate the so-called central flows, that is, the flows through the *foramen ovale*, the *ductus arteriosus*, and the *aortic isthmus*. Table 7-2 illustrates how these calculations are done. Although the principle of the calculations is sound, there is considerable error in measuring the relatively small differences in microsphere concentrations between ascending and descending aorta and between ascending aorta and pulmonary artery. The same concerns apply if the oxygen content in these three vessels is used to calculate the relative contribution of *ductus arteriosus* and isthmus flow to abdominal (descending) aorta flow as originally suggested by Dawes *et al.* (11). For example, in nine fetal sheep we have studied, the mean *ductus arteriosus : abdominal aorta* flow ratio was 0.74 ± 0.1 as calculated by means of the microsphere data and 0.66 ± 0.07 as calculated by means of the oxygen content data. To circumvent this difficulty, Anderson *et al.* (2) have combined the microsphere technique with a direct measurement of right ventricular output by means of a flow meter on the pulmonary artery. Their results are presented in Table 7-3 together with the results from our laboratory which are based on oxygen and microsphere data alone. It is important to note that the fetal right : left ventricle output ratio has been a matter of controversy, with estimates ranging from 0.82 to 2.0. The most recent evidence seems to indicate that right ventricular output exceeds left ventricular output. However, there is no reason to assume that the relative contributions of each ventricle to cardiac output is a constant value.

Early studies employing microsphere methodology demonstrated conclusively the salient feature of fetal cardiac output distribution; namely, that the placenta receives approximately 40% of the combined output of

Table 7-2

Calculation of Ductus Arteriosus Flow (F_D), Right Ventricular
Output (V_R), Flow through the Aortic Isthmus (F_I), Left Ventricular
Output (V_L), and Flow through the Foramen Ovale (F_{FO})

Given:
  Combined cardiac output (CO)
    Flow to heart and upper body (F_{HU})
    Flow to lower body and placenta (F_{LP})
    Flow to lungs (f)
  Concentration of microspheres in
    Pulmonary artery (M_{pa})
    Ascending aorta (M_{as})
    Abdominal aorta (M_{ab})

The quantity of spheres carried by the ductus arteriosus flow ($M_{pa} \times F_D$) mixes with the quantity carried by the flow through the aortic isthmus ($M_{as} \times F_I$) to form the quantity carried to the lower body and placenta ($M_{ab} \times F_{LP}$):

$$(M_{pa} \times F_D) + (M_{as} \times F_I) = M_{ab} \times F_{LP} \tag{1}$$

Since

$$F_D + F_I = F_{LP} \tag{2}$$

$$F_D = \left(\frac{M_{as} - M_{ab}}{M_{as} - M_{pa}}\right) F_{LP} \tag{3}$$

Also,

$$V_R = F_D + f \tag{4}$$

$$F_I = F_{LP} - F_D \tag{5}$$

$$V_L = F_I + F_{HU} \tag{6}$$

$$F_{FO} = V_L - f \tag{7}$$

the fetal heart, whereas the lungs receive a small fraction of it, usually less than 10% (Figure 7-3). Subsequent studies have focused upon defining the factors which may alter the magnitude and distribution of fetal cardiac output.

In comparing lamb fetuses at different gestational ages, Rudolph and Heymann (37) observed a relatively constant cardiac output per kilogram of fetal body weight. They also observed age related changes in distribution of cardiac output, with the placenta receiving a larger fraction and organs such as gut and lungs receiving a smaller fraction of cardiac output at mid-gestation than at term (Figure 7-3). The observations in early fetal life, however, were not in unstressed, chronic preparations. As discussed in Chapter 6, there are striking changes in the distribution of fetal cardiac output with acute hypoxia.

Table 7-3

Ventricular Outputs and Central Blood Flows in the Fetal Lamb Expressed as Percentage of Combined Ventricular Output[a]

Source	Right ventricle	Left ventricle	Lungs	Ductus arteriosus	Foramen ovale	Aortic isthmus	Heart + upper body	Lower body + placenta
Anderson et al. (2)	59.8 ± 7.8	40.2 ± 8.2	6.2 ± 1.5	53.6 ± 8.3	34.0 ± 7.8	12.4 ± 5.5	27.7	66.1
Sheldon et al. (40)	50.4[b]	49.6[b]	4.3	46.1[b]	45.3[b]	19.8[b]	29.8 ± 1.2	65.9 ± 1.2

[a] Values given as mean ± SEM.
[b] Based on the estimate that the *ductus arteriosus* : lower body + placenta flow ratio is 0.7.

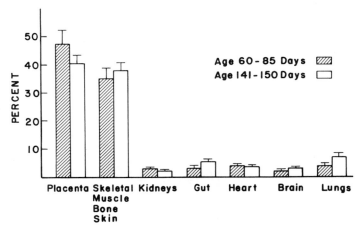

Figure 7-3:   Percent distribution (± SEM) of cardiac output in the ovine fetus at two gestational ages (37).

BLOOD VOLUME AND ARTERIAL PRESSURE

The fetus has a relatively low blood pressure and a large blood volume. The normal arterial blood pressure of fetal lambs in the last month of gestation is approximately 42 Torr, that is, 42 Torr higher than the amniotic pressure. The pressure in the amniotic cavity is the appropriate reference for fetal blood pressure measurements because it represents the pressure over the surface of the fetal body and umbilical cord. Clearly, amniotic pressure will vary depending upon uterine tone and maternal intraabdominal pressure. Experiments in exteriorized fetuses have suggested that fetal blood pressure may be substantially lower earlier in gestation, in the 20–30 Torr range. It would be interesting to verify these observations in chronic preparations.

The blood volume in the fetal circulation has been measured in sheep using the simultaneous injection of ^{51}Cr labeled red cells and albumin tagged with ^{125}I (8). In fetuses with body weight ranging between 1.33 and 5.42 kg, blood volume (in milliliters) was related to weight (in kilograms) by the regression equation:

$$\text{Blood volume} = 136.7 \text{ wt} - 8.1 \quad (R = 0.82)$$

(Note that fetal weight does not include the weight of the placenta.) The equation suggests a simple proportionality between the blood volume of the fetal circulation and the fetal weight. Early observations by Barcroft (4), however, had indicated that the blood volume in the placental vascular bed of sheep does not increase in the last 50 days of gestation and remains approximately equal to 100 ml. This observation is consistent with the fact that the placenta is not increasing in size over this time period as well. Thus, the volume of the fetal circulation probably has two components: a component (placental blood volume) which grows at a slow rate in the second half of pregnancy and a component which increases rapidly in relation to fetal weight (blood within the fetal body).

HEART RATE AND STROKE VOLUME
IN RELATION TO BODY WEIGHT AND OXYGEN DEMANDS

Fetal heart rate has been measured under normal physiologic conditions in humans, sheep and guinea pigs. We believe that from a basic physiological viewpoint the most interesting aspect to emerge from these studies has been the observation that the heart rate of immature fetuses tends to be the same among different mammals, irrespective of their large differences in body size (30). This contrasts to the inverse relationship of heart rate to body weight in adult mammals (Figure 7-4) (17). In adult mammals that differ in body mass by one or more orders of magnitude, heart weight tends to be a constant fraction of body weight. This appears to be true for fetuses as well (Table 7-4). As a consequence in both adult and fetal mammals, stroke volume tends to be proportional to body weight. Since stroke volume × heart rate = cardiac output, it follows that fetal cardiac output per kilogram body weight (that is, weight-specific

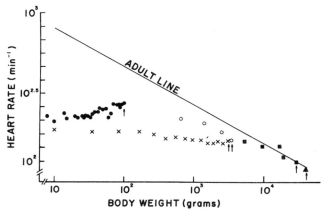

Figure 7-4:   Logarithmic plot of heart rate versus body weight in fetuses of different species. Guinea pig fetus, ● (30); human fetus, X (18); ovine fetus, ○ (42); bovine fetus, ■ (34); and equine fetus, ▲ (30). The "adult line" represents the relationship of heart rate to body mass in adult mammals (30).

Table 7-4

Fetal Heart Weight : Body Weight Ratios in Different Species[a]

Species	Ratio ($\times 100$)	Reference
Rat	0.65	41
Guinea pig	0.52	30
Rhesus monkey	0.65	26
Pig	0.65	44
Sheep	0.64	Unpublished data
Human	0.65	16

[a] All data refer to fetuses close to term.

cardiac output) must be similar among fetuses of different sizes and species. In turn, similarity of weight-specific cardiac output implies a similarity in the weight-specific oxygen consumption rate because the main function of cardiac output is to provide oxygen to the tissues. It is important to emphasize that comparative studies of fetal metabolism on the one hand (Chapter 3) and fetal heart rate on the other are mutually supportive evidence showing that the intensity of oxidative metabolism expressed per unit body weight is approximately the same among the immature fetuses of small and large mammals. Comparative observations of fetal heart rate in different species are particularly important because such data can be obtained under normal physiologic conditions and they include reliable data about the human fetus.

An interesting consequence of the independence of fetal heart rate from body weight in the immature fetus is that, as gestation progresses, fetal heart rate changes in opposite directions in small and large mammals. In the fetal guinea pig normal heart rate is quite stable at 212 ± 3 beats/min in the 38–50 day gestation period, a time when fetal weight increases from 8 to 30 (Figure 7-5) (30). However, after 50 days gestation, heart rate begins to increase and attains a value of 259 ± 5 beats/min in the last days before birth. From the viewpoint of adult physiology, the increasing fetal heart rate coincident with an increase of body weight from 30 to 100 is paradoxical. However, its functional meaning becomes evident once we realize that the heart rate and cardiac output of a mature fetal guinea pig are much less than the heart rate and cardiac output necessary for a free postnatal existence. If the heart rate of adult mammals is used as the standard for full adaptation to extrauterine life, the appropriate heart rate for a newborn guinea pig that weighs 100g should be approximately 430 beats/min rather than the 212 beats/min of the immature fetus. From this

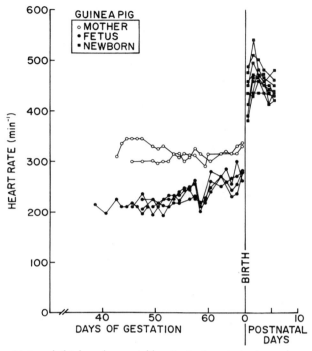

Figure 7-5: Maternal, fetal, and neonatal heart rates in guinea pigs under normal physiologic conditions (30).

viewpoint, it is understandable that the fetal guinea pig should begin to increase its heart rate in preparation for birth. Note, however, that the biggest increase happens after birth as the newborn rapidly adapts to the new environment by acquiring a heart rate in the 400–500 beats/min range during the first few days of neonatal life.

In contrast to the guinea pig, the maturational changes of fetal heart rate in the ovine (42) and bovine (34) fetuses are characterized by a decrease of fetal heart rate (Figure 7-4). This is probably because the production of a mature newborn of large size involves the production of a large skeletal and muscle mass, which requires less oxygen per unit weight than the viscera. Since metabolic rate per kilogram may be falling, there follows a corresponding reduction in heart rate.

To analyze the performance of the fetal heart, it is instructive to compare the relationship of heart rate to oxygen demands in fetal and adult mammals. In adults at rest, both heart rate and weight-specific oxygen consumption vary inversely to body weight, and the negative exponents of the allometric equations that relate both of these rates to weight are virtually equal. This observation implies that in adult mammals the number of heart beats per milliliter (STP) of oxygen consumed per unit body weight is approximately constant. From the data reviewed by Gunther (17), one can calculate that the value of this constant is 24 beats/ml_{STP} oxygen. If the heart rate of a 3-kg sheep fetus (160 beats/min) is divided by its weight-specific oxygen consumption rate (7 ml_{STP}/kg/min), one obtains a similar value of 23 beats/ml_{STP} oxygen. This is a surprising result because the fetus lives in a state of physiologic hypoxia that requires a relatively high cardiac output. In a 3-kg adult mammal at rest, the biventricular cardiac output : oxygen consumption ratio is approximately 40 ml/ml_{STP}, whereas in a 3-kg sheep fetus the same ratio is approximately 70 ml/ml_{STP}. Since there is no evidence that fetal heart rate is disproportionately high with respect to oxygen demands, it appears that the main adaptation of cardiac function to the physiologic demands of fetal life is a larger stroke volume. At mid-gestation in sheep, fetal heart size is relatively large in comparison to body size. Later in pregnancy, however, the heart : body mass ratio becomes virtually identical to that of adult mammals. This indicates that, in the mature fetus, stroke volume is large in relation to heart size.

REGULATION OF FETAL CIRCULATION

The regulation of fetal circulation has certain unique characteristics as well as similarities with postnatal regulation. Foremost among the conditions that require a special regulatory arrangement in fetal life are the presence of the umbilical circulation and the shunting of blood across the lungs via the *ductus arteriosus* and the *foramen ovale*.

Several studies have shown that fetal venous and arterial pressures as well as cardiac output can be readily decreased by the rapid withdrawal of blood, whereas the rapid infusion of blood or saline causes a substantial increase of venous and arterial pressures without marked changes in cardiac output and heart rate (15). These observations indicate that under normal physiologic conditions the stroke work of the fetal heart is near the maximum of a cardiac function curve (Figure 7-6) (15), and they support the concept that the fetus maintains a high cardiac output by maintaining a large stroke volume.

Both the umbilical and fetal systemic circulations are essential parts of the oxygen delivery system from placenta to fetal tissues. Intuitively, the fraction of cardiac output perfusing the placenta must be balanced against the fraction perfusing the fetal body to attain optimal delivery of the

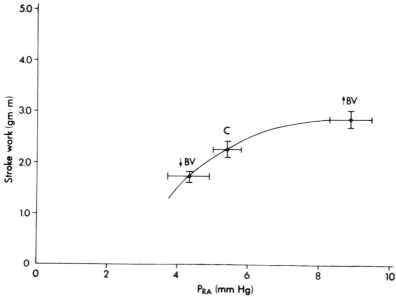

Figure 7-6: Relationship of biventricular stroke work to right atrial pressures (P_{RA}) in the fetal lamb under control conditions (C), after increasing fetal blood volume by 10% (↑ BV), and after withdrawal of 10% of fetal blood (↓ BV). The measurements were made within 15 min of blood volume changes (15).

available oxygen. Figure 7-7 presents a model of the fetal circulation to assist us in assessing this intuition quantitatively. The model is much simpler than the actual circulation, but adequate for the purpose at hand. Umbilical and systemic venous returns mix to form the output of the fetal heart. The blood ejected by the fetal heart is divided into two blood flows: the flow through the umbilical circulation and the systemic blood flow. The model predicts that, for any given set of values for fetal cardiac output, fetal oxygen requirement, and umbilical venous oxygen content, there is an optimal umbilical blood flow at which systemic oxygen delivery is maximal (Figure 7-8). With a decrease in blood oxygenation, oxygen delivery is favored by a moderate increase in the fraction of cardiac output perfusing the umbilical circulation.

It is noteworthy that the optimal umbilical flow : cardiac output ratio predicted by the model for a normal level of oxygenation is within the range of experimental values. The mechanisms by which the fetus maintains the appropriate balance between placental and somatic circulations are not well understood. The umbilical circulation is not innervated, but its resistance can be increased by several vasoactive substances (e.g.,

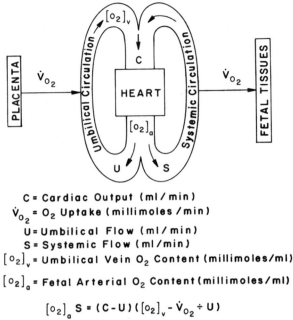

C = Cardiac Output (ml/min)
$\dot{V}_{O_2}$ = O_2 Uptake (millimoles/min)
U = Umbilical Flow (ml/min)
S = Systemic Flow (ml/min)
$[O_2]_v$ = Umbilical Vein O_2 Content (millimoles/ml)

$[O_2]_a$ = Fetal Arterial O_2 Content (millimoles/ml)

$$[O_2]_a \, S = (C - U)([O_2]_v - \dot{V}_{O_2} \div U)$$

Figure 7-7: Mathematical model of the fetal circulation showing the relationship of fetal systemic arterial oxygen delivery (i.e., the arterial oxygen content × systemic blood flow product) to fetal cardiac output, umbilical blood flow, umbilical venous oxygen content, and fetal oxygen consumption (31).

angiotensin II, several prostaglandins, and bradykinin) which presumably play some role in this regulation (32).

Under normal physiologic conditions both fetal blood pressure and heart rate vary spontaneously with a coefficient of variation which is similar to that of maternal pressure and heart rate under resting conditions. This variability can be decreased by the fetal injection of hexamethonium, a ganglionic blocker which also decreases mean fetal blood pressure and heart rate (Figure 7-9) (27). In contrast, the variability of fetal blood pressure can be increased by sinoaortic denervation (19, 45). These results seem in conflict with studies indicating that the increase in fetal blood pressure required to elicit a baroreflex is quite large and apparently outside the boundaries of normal fetal blood pressure variability (11). The reasons for this conflict are obscure.

In the fetal lamb the carotid chemoreceptors appear to be quiescent and rather insensitive to hypoxic stimulation. However, Dawes et al. (10) showed that the aortic chemoreceptors can be stimulated by fetal asphyxia and cause vasoconstriction in the hind limbs.

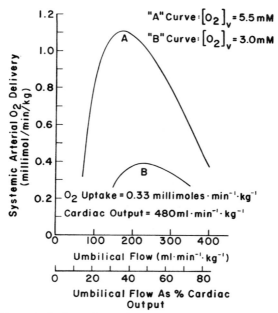

Figure 7-8: Theoretical relationship of fetal systemic arterial oxygen delivery to umbilical blood flow at normal values of fetal cardiac output and oxygen uptake and at two different levels of umbilical venous oxygen content.

The influence of vagal and adrenergic innervation on the fetal heart has been clearly demonstrated by observing the effects of atropine (parasympathetic blocker) and propranolol (β-adrenergic blocker) on fetal heart rate at different gestational ages (42). Vagal inhibition increases with advancing gestation, representing the principal mechanism by which the heart rate of fetal lambs declines as their body weight increases. Since a growth-related decrease of heart rate is not present in small mammals, it is unwarranted to assume that the age-related changes in autonomic control observed in sheep are a general characteristic of fetal growth.

Several hormones and vasoactive substances contribute to the regulation of the fetal circulation, both under normal conditions and in response to emergency situations such as hypoxia and hemorrhage (3, 32). Hormonal regulation of the vascular system may be particularly important in the fetus because almost half of fetal cardiac output perfuses the umbilical vasculature which is not under neural control. A vasoactive peptide (vasotocin) which is present in early fetal life has been described, but its physiologic role remains conjectural (39). The roles of vasopressin, the angiotensin-renin system, catecholamines, and prostaglandins in regulating the fetal circulation have been studied by several investigators. Vaso-

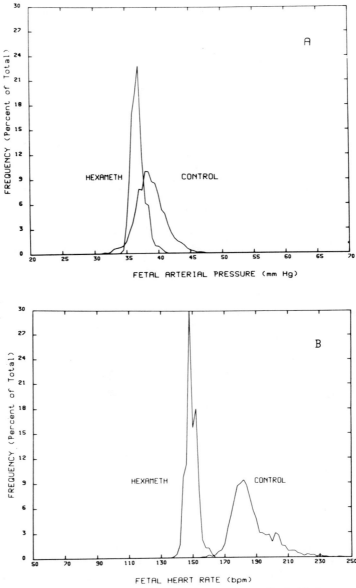

Figure 7-9: Example of the effect of hexamethonium, a ganglionic blocker, on mean and variability of fetal blood pressure and heart rate (27).

pressin (ADH) is normally present in fetal blood at concentrations which are similar to those in adult blood. When infused at a low dose into fetal lambs, it has no detectable effect on blood pressure, but does decrease urinary output markedly coincident with an increase in urine osmolarity (28). At higher doses it increases blood pressure by reducing blood flow to the gut and carcass, and it increases the umbilical flow : somatic flow ratio (22). The plasma concentration of fetal vasopressin increases in response to severe hypoxia (38), to the rapid withdrawal of blood (35), and to the infusion of hypertonic NaCl (43). Some investigators have suggested that vasopressin may regulate the flux of water across the placenta by modifying placental conductance to osmotic flow, but the evidence supporting this hypothesis is largely indirect.

In chronic fetal lamb preparations, plasma renin activity is relatively high and can be increased or decreased by reducing or increasing, respectively, fetal blood volume (32). The fetal infusion of saralasin, an angiotensin II competitive inhibitor, causes a small but significant decrease in fetal arterial pressure (20). The fetal infusion of angiotensin II at doses that reproduce the plasma levels observed in response to moderate hemorrhage induces an increase of blood pressure and a constriction of the umbilical vascular bed with a reduction of the umbilical : somatic flow ratio (21).

Under normal physiologic conditions, the fetal plasma level of catecholamines is quite low. However, severe hypoxia increases the plasma concentrations of both norepinephrine and epinephrine markedly (23). The main source of plasma epinephrine is the fetal adrenal gland, whereas plasma norepinephrine has multiple sources. The epinephrine response to hypoxia is more pronounced in the mature fetus, probably reflecting developmental changes of the adrenal gland. Norepinephrine increases the resistance of the somatic vascular bed, whereas it has little or no effect on the resistance of the umbilical circulation (29). Consequently, norepinephrine tends to increase the umbilical : somatic blood flow ratio.

Prostaglandins play an important regulatory role on the *ductus arteriosus*. Indomethacin (a prostaglandin synthesis inhibitor) causes a constriction of the *ductus arteriosus* in fetal sheep and an increased pressure difference between the pulmonary artery and the aorta (6, 7). The infusion of prostaglandin E_2 (PGE_2) promptly dilates the *ductus*. It is not clear whether the patency of the *ductus arteriosus* depends on the local production of prostaglandins or, in part, on prostaglandins produced by the placenta and carried to the *ductus* via the fetal circulation. The level of PGE_2 in fetal blood is relatively high, thus supporting the notion that some prostaglandins play the role of circulatory hormones in fetal life (6).

Oxygen is an important regulator of the fetal circulation. It influences the distribution of fetal cardiac output both by having a local effect on the circulation of different organs and indirectly via chemoreceptor stimulation. Three distinct patterns of response to oxygen have been identified in different fetal organs (33).

Type I Response

This response is characteristic of the heart, central nervous system, and adrenals. Local mechanisms of circulatory control in the heart and central nervous system markedly increase the rate of perfusion as arterial oxygen content decreases secondary to a decrease of arterial P_{O_2}. Figure 7-10 presents data for the coronary and cerebral circulations, demonstrating that the inverse relationship of coronary and cerebral blood flow to arterial oxygen content is hyperbolic and that fetal cerebral vasodilatation is stimulated by hypercapnea as well. Because of these relationships of flow to oxygen content, the supply of oxygen to heart and brain (i.e., the product of blood flow × arterial oxygen content) tends to remain at a normal level during moderate hypoxia. However, the maintenance of a

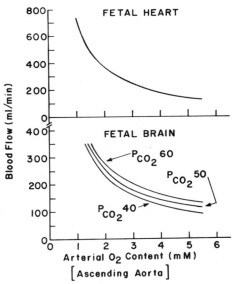

Figure 7-10: Upper panel: Relationship of coronary flow to arterial oxygen content in the lamb fetus. Curve constructed from data by Peeters et al. (33). Lower panel: Relationship of cerebral blood flow to arterial oxygen content and P_{CO_2} in the lamb fetus. Curves constructed from data by Jones et al. (25).

normal level of oxygen supply while arterial P_{O_2} is below normal cannot prevent a decrease of P_{O_2} within the tissue capillaries. To benefit from a relatively normal oxygen delivery rate in the presence of a low capillary P_{O_2}, a tissue must have intrinsic properties which favor the diffusion of oxygen from erythrocytes to mitochondria, such as a large capillary surface and a short distance between cells and capillaries. This is probably true for the fetal brain and heart. It has been shown that fetal cerebral oxygen uptake can remain at its normal level even when the venous blood in the sagittal sinus has a P_{O_2} as low as 9 Torr and an oxygen content which is less than 0.5 mM (24). Similar observations have been made for the fetal heart (14). In addition to the central nervous system and heart, the adrenal glands respond to even moderate hypoxia with a large increase of blood flow.

Type II Response

The blood flow to kidneys, gut, and the nonvisceral parts of the fetus (skeletal muscle, skin, and bones, sometimes referred to as the fetal carcass) either remains constant or increases moderately as fetal oxygen-

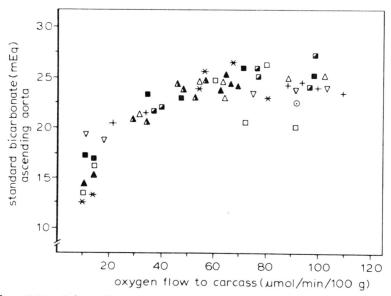

Figure 7-11:   Relationship between the standard bicarbonate of fetal arterial blood and the oxygen flow to the fetal carcass. The oxygen flow was calculated by multiplying arterial oxygen content times the blood flow to the fetal carcass (33).

ation begins to decrease, but then decreases precipitously in severe acute hypoxia. This complex response is due to the action of two sets of regulatory mechanisms with opposite effects: a set of local mechanisms which tend to increase local blood flow in response to hypoxia and a set of systemic mechanisms triggered by chemoreceptor stimulation which tend to decrease blood flow. The metabolic acidosis that develops in severe fetal hypoxia is associated with an inadequate supply of oxygen to the fetal carcass (Figure 7-11). The vasoconstriction of the gastrointestinal tract and kidneys in response to hypoxia may have considerable clinical significance. It is well recognized that a renal injury manifested by oliguria, hematuria, and proteinuria is not at all infrequent following perinatal asphyxia. In addition, perinatal asphyxia has been associated with an increased frequency of necrotizing enterocolitis. The fact that the gastrointestinal tract may vasoconstrict in response to hypoxia suggests caution in attempting oral feedings soon after a perinatal asphyxial episode in newborn infants.

Type III Response

Blood flow to the fetal lungs is unique in showing a positive correlation with arterial P_{O_2}. Fetal pulmonary blood flow increases when fetal P_{O_2} is increased by administration of oxygen to the mother and decreases in response to a decrease in P_{O_2}. The constrictive effect of hypoxia on the pulmonary circulation is thought to play an important role in the etiology of the so-called persistent fetal circulation syndrome and pulmonary hypertension of the neonate.

The effect of oxygen on pulmonary blood flow suggests the attractive hypothesis that the low P_{O_2} of fetal blood plays an important physiologic role, being the agent that maintains the high resistance of the fetal pulmonary circulation. However, there are two considerations making us cautious about accepting this hypothesis. First, oxygen is only one of several factors that can influence the tone of the fetal pulmonary vasculature. Acetylcholine, histamine, bradykinin, and prostaglandin E have all been shown to decrease pulmonary vascular resistance at relatively low doses (32). Second, most of the studies regarding the vascular resistance of the fetal pulmonary circulation have been carried out over relatively short time periods and may not be relevant to chronic regulation. Experiments by Accurso *et al.* in our laboratory (1) indicate that the dilatation of the pulmonary vascular bed caused by an increase in fetal pulmonary arterial P_{O_2} is a transient response, with pulmonary flow returning to control values after approximately 2 hr exposure to the higher P_{O_2}.

REFERENCES

1. Accurso, F.J., Alpert, B., Petersen, R.G. and Meschia, G. (1986). *Time-dependent response of fetal pulmonary blood flow to an increase in fetal oxygen tension.* Respiratory Physiology **63**, 43–52.
2. Anderson, D.F., Bissonnette, J.M., Faber, J.J. and Thornburg, K.L. (1981). *Central shunt flows and pressures in the mature fetal lamb.* American Journal of Physiology **241**, H60–H66.
3. Assali, N.S., Brinkman, C.R. III, Woods, J.R. Jr., et al. (1977). *Development of neurohumoral control of fetal, neonatal, and adult cardiovascular functions.* American Journal of Obstetrics and Gynecology **129**, 748–758.
4. Barcroft, J. (1947). "Researches on Prenatal Life," Thomas, Springfield, Illinois.
5. Born, G.V.R., Dawes, G.S., Mott, J.C. and Widdicombe, J.G. (1954). *Changes in the heart and lungs at birth.* Cold Spring Harbor Symposia in Quarterly Biology **19**, 102–107.
6. Challis, J.R.G., Hart, I., Lotis, T.M., Mitchell, M.D., Jenkin, G., Robinson, J.S. and Thorburn, G.D. (1978). *Prostaglandins in the sheep fetus: Implications for fetal function.* Advances in Prostaglandin Thromboxane Research **4**, 115–132.
7. Clyman, R.I. and Heymann, M.A. (1981). *Pharmacology of the ductus arteriosus.* Pediatric Clinics of North America **28**, 77–93.
8. Creasy, R.K., Drost, M., Green, M.V. and Morris, J.A. (1970). *Determination of fetal, placental and neonatal blood volumes in the sheep.* Circulation Research **27**, 487–494.
9. Dawes, G.S., Mott, J.C. and Widdicombe, J.G. (1954). *The foetal circulation in the lamb.* Journal of Physiology **126**, 563–587.
10. Dawes, G.S., Lewis, B.V., Milligan, J.E., Roach, M.R. and Talner, N.S. (1968). *Vasomotor responses in the hind limbs of foetal and newborn lambs to asphyxia and aortic chemoreceptor stimulation.* Journal of Physiology **195**, 55–81.
11. Dawes, G.S., Johnston, B.M. and Walker, D.W. (1980). *Relationship of arterial pressure and heart rate in fetal, newborn and adult sheep.* Journal of Physiology **309**, 405–417.
12. Edelstone, D.I., Rudolph, A.M. and Heymann, M.A. (1978). *Liver and ductus venosus blood flows in the fetal lamb in utero.* Circulation Research **42**, 426–433.
13. Edelstone, D.I. and Rudolph, A.M. (1979). *Preferential streaming of ductus venosus blood to the brain and heart in fetal lambs.* American Journal of Physiology **237**, H724–H729.
14. Fisher, D.J., Heymann, M.A. and Rudolph, A.M. (1982). *Fetal myocardial oxygen and carbohydrate metabolism in sustained hypoxemia in utero.* American Journal of Physiology **243**, H959–H963.
15. Gilbert, R.D. (1980). *Control of fetal cardiac output during changes in blood volume.* American Journal of Physiology **238**, H80–H86.
16. Gruenwald, P. (1963). *Chronic fetal distress and placental insufficiency.* Biology of the Neonate **5**, 215–265.
17. Gunther, B. (1975). *Dimensional analysis and theory of biological similarity.* Physiologic Reviews **55**, 659–699.
18. Ibarra-Polo, A.A., Guiloff, E., Gomez-Rogers, C. (1972). *Fetal heart rate throughout pregnancy.* American Journal of Obstetrics and Gynecology **113**, 814–818.
19. Itskovitz, J., LaGamma, E.F. and Rudolph, A.M. (1983). *Baroreflex control of the circulation in chronically instrumental fetal lambs.* Circulation Research **52**, 589–596.
20. Iwamoto, H.S. and Rudolph, A.M. (1979). *Effects of endogenous angiotensin II on the fetal circulation.* Journal of Developmental Physiology **1**, 283–293.

21. Iwamoto, H.S. and Rudolph, A.M. (1981). *Effects of angiotensin II on the blood flow and its distribution in fetal lambs.* Circulation Research **48**, 183–189.

22. Iwamoto, H.S., Rudolph, A.M., Keil, L.C.S. and Heymann, M.A. (1979). *Hemodynamic responses of the sheep fetus to vasopressin infusion.* Circulation Research **44**, 430–436.

23. Jones, C.T. and Robinson, R.O. (1975). *Plasma catecholamines in foetal and adult sheep.* Journal of Physiology (London) **248**, 15–53.

24. Jones, M.D. Jr., Sheldon, R.E., Peeters, L.L.H., Meschia, G., Battaglia, F.C. and Makowski, E.L. (1977). *Fetal cerebral oxygen consumption at different levels of oxygenation.* Journal of Applied Physiology **43**, 1080–1084.

25. Jones, M.D. Jr., Sheldon, R.E., Peeters, L.L.H., Makowski, E.L. and Meschia, G. (1978). *Regulation of cerebral blood flow in the ovine fetus.* American Journal of Physiology **235**, H162–H166.

26. Kerr, G.R., Kennan, A.L., Wasiman, H.A. and Allen, J.R. (1969). *Growth and development of the fetal rhesus monkey. I. Physical growth.* Growth **33**, 201–213.

27. Lawler, F.H. and Brace, R.A. (1982). *Fetal and maternal arterial pressures and heart rates: histograms, correlations, and rhythms.* American Journal of Physiology **243**, R433–R444.

28. Lingwood, B., Hardy, J.J., Horacek, I., McPhee, M.L., Scoggins, B.A. and Wintour, E.M. (1978). *The effects of antidiuretic hormone on urine flow and composition in the chronically cannulated ovine fetus.* Quarterly Journal of Experimental Physiology and Cognitive Medical Sciences **63**, 315–330.

29. Lorijn, R.H.W. and Longo, L.D. (1980). *Norepinephrine elevation in the fetal lamb: Oxygen consumption and cardiac output.* American Journal of Physiology **239**, R115–R122.

30. Meier, P.R., Manchester, D.K., Battaglia, F.C. and Meschia, G. (1983). *Fetal heart rate in relation to body mass.* Proceedings of the Society for Experimental Biology and Medicine **172**, 107–110.

31. Meschia, G. (1985). *Safety margin of fetal oxygenation.* Journal of Reproductive Medicine **30**, 308–311.

32. Mott, J.C. and Walker, D.W. (1983). *Neural and endocrine regulation of circulation in the fetus and newborn.* In "Handbook of Physiology: The Cardiovascular System," (J.T. Shepherd and F.M. Abboud, eds.), Section 2, Volume III, pp. 837–883, American Physiologic Society, Bethesda, Maryland.

33. Peeters, L.L.H., Sheldon, R.E., Jones, M.D. Jr., Makowski, E.L. and Meschia, G. (1979). *Blood flow to fetal organs as a function of arterial oxygen content.* American Journal of Obstetrics and Gynecology **135**, 637–646.

34. Reeves, J.T., Daoud, F.S. and Gentry, M. (1972). *Growth of the fetal calf and its arterial pressure, blood gases, and hematologic data.* Journal of Applied Physiology **32**, 240–244.

35. Robillard, J.E., Weitzman, R.E., Fisher, D.A. and Smith, F.G. (1979). *The dynamics of vasopressin release and blood volume regulation during fetal hemorrhage in the lamb fetus.* Pediatric Research **13**, 606–610.

36. Rudolph, A.M. and Heymann, M.A. (1967). *The circulation of the fetus in utero: Methods for studying distribution of blood flow.* Circulation Research **21**, 163–184.

37. Rudolph, A.M. and Heymann, M.A. (1970). *Circulatory changes during growth in the fetal lamb.* Circulation Research **26**, 289–299.

38. Rurak, D.W. (1978). *Plasma vasopressin levels during hypoxaemia and the cardiovascular effects of exogenous vasopressin in foetal and adult sheep.* Journal of Physiology (London) **277**, 341–357.

39. Sawyer, W.H. (1977). *Evolution of neurohypophyseal hormones and their receptors.* Federation Proceedings **36**, 1842–1847.

40. Sheldon, R.E., Peeters, L.L.H., Jones, M.D. Jr., Makowski, E.L. and Meschia, G. (1979). *Redistribution of cardiac output and oxygen delivery in the hypoxemic fetal lamb.* American Journal of Obstetrics and Gynecology **135**, 1071–1078.

41. Sikov, M.R. and Thomas, J.M. (1970). *Prenatal growth of the rat.* Growth **34**, 1–14.

42. Walker, A.M., Cannata, J., Dowling, M.H., Ritchie, B. and Maloney, J.E. (1978). *Sympathetic and parasympathetic control of heart rate in unanaesthetized fetal and newborn lambs.* Biology of the Neonate **33**, 135–143.

43. Weitzman, R.E., Fisher, D.A., Robillard, J., Erenberg, A., Kennedy, R. and Smith, F. (1978). *Arginine vasopressin response to an osmotic stimulus in the fetal sheep.* Pediatric Research **12**, 35–38.

44. Widdowson, E.M. (1971). *Intrauterine growth retardation in the pig.* Biology of the Neonate **19**, 329–340.

45. Yardley, R.W., Bowes, G., Wilkinson, M., Cannata, J.P., Maloney, J.E., Ritchie, B.C. and Walker, A.M. (1983). *Increased arterial pressure variability after arterial baroreceptor denervation in fetal lambs.* Circulation Research **52**, 580–588.

8

Uteroplacental Blood Flow

CHRONIC CHANGES DURING PREGNANCY

Pregnancy requires an increased rate of uterine perfusion. In sheep, uterine blood flow and its two major components (myoendometrial and placental cotyledonary flow) have been measured during the estrous cycle as well as throughout pregnancy (Table 8-1) (19, 20, 47). During the estrous cycle uterine blood flow waxes and wanes in response to hormonal stimulation and attains a maximal value at estrous (19). Following insemination, uterine blood flow decreases and continues to decrease for approximately 16 days (20). This is the preimplantation stage of embryonic development. Between days 16 and 50, the fetal chorion becomes attached to the uterine mucosa, the placental cotyledons are formed, and the rate of perfusion of the uterus begins to increase both absolutely and in relation to tissue weight and tissue oxygen consumption. At day 38, for example, uterine blood flow is approximately 900 ml/kg of combined myoendometrial, cotyledonary, and fetal weight and the coefficient of oxygen extraction is about 10% (Figure 8-1). In the next stage of development, which extends approximately from 50 to 90 days, the placental cotyledons grow to their maximum size and become the largest component of the uterine mass. In this period cotyledonary flow increases to approximately 300 ml/min and becomes the larger fraction (approximately 65%) of uterine blood flow. In the last 2 months of pregnancy placental weight decreases, but placental blood flow continues to in-

Table 8-1

Uterine, Placental, and Fetal Growth in Sheep and Concurrent Changes in Rate of Uterine Perfusion[a]

Stage	Fetal age (days)	Type[b]	Fetus[c]	Weight (g)		Blood flow (ml/min)		
				Myometrium and endometrium	Placental cotyledons	Myometrium and endometrium	Placental cotyledons	Total uterine flow
Nonpregnant ovariectomized	—	—	—	71	7[d]	18	7[d]	25
Stage II	38	T	3.4	109	8	81	31	112
	47	S	13.3	145	53	125	45	170
Stage III	57	T	78	215	341	147	259	406
	60	T	137	295	479	195	271	466
	64	S	92	184	311	125	161	286
	67	T	188	276	570	162	326	488
	74	S	186	270	732	100	316	416
	78	T	188	338	605	198	255	453
	85	T	513	425	817	152	307	458
Stage IV	98	S	935	363	295	99	443	542
	98	T	1003	342	799	143	578	721
	112	T	2795	437	597	143	573	716
	113	T	2750	546	529	179	615	794
	119	S	1800	341	356	102	1047	1149
	120	S	1735	407	348	77	437	514
	127	T	2380	474	269	158	849	1007
	131	S	3150	475	193	215	535	750
	131	S	2950	462	296	166	839	1005
	132	T	5085	687	676	225	1101	1326
	133	T	5175	677	515	176	1246	1522
	134	T	4570	548	421	175	1565	1740
	138	S	2480	311	189	222	492	714
	139	S	4285	649	428	192	1323	1515
	140	S	4715	627	499	275	1543	1818

[a] From Rosenfeld et al. (49).

[b] Data are from 13 twin (T) and 11 single (S) pregnancies.

[c] Data for twins are combined weight.

[d] Data for caruncular tissue.

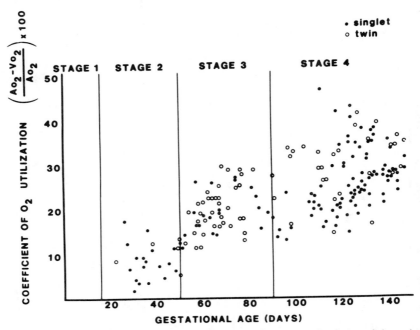

Figure 8-1: Coefficient of oxygen utilization across the uterine circulation of sheep from early pregnancy to term (33, 34).

crease, normally attaining values from 1 to 2 liters/min. From 120 days to term cotyledonary blood flow is usually 80–90% of uterine blood flow (Figure 8-2).

The increase in uterine blood flow during ovine pregnancy does not match closely the growth in oxygen demands by placenta and fetus as demonstrated by the observation that the coefficient of oxygen utilization across the sheep uterus becomes larger with advancing gestation (Figure 8-1). Similar observations have been made in other species with different placental types. The data for the rabbit uterine circulation are shown in Figure 8-3 (37). In both the guinea pig and the rabbit the coefficient of extraction for oxygen by the pregnant uterus is remarkably higher by the end of gestation (60–70%) than in sheep (20–40%). However, the basic observation that the increased oxygen requirements of the growing fetus are met by both an increase in uterine blood flow and by an increasing oxygen extraction is true in all three species. Such observations have been the basis for the theory that in the last part of gestation the fetus tends to outgrow the ability of maternal placental blood flow to provide oxygen. In a famous analogy, Barcroft (2) compared the growing fetus to

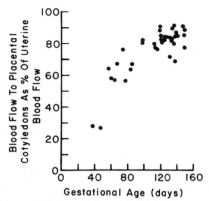

Figure 8-2:   Blood flow to the placental cotyledons of sheep expressed as a percentage of total uterine blood flow from early pregnancy to term. Figure constructed from data by Rosenfeld (48).

a mountain climber. In climbing to higher elevations, the climber is exposed to a progressively decreasing P_{O_2}. Similarly, the growing fetus would be exposed to a progressively decreasing P_{O_2} as it extracts progressively larger quantities of oxygen from the maternal blood that perfuses

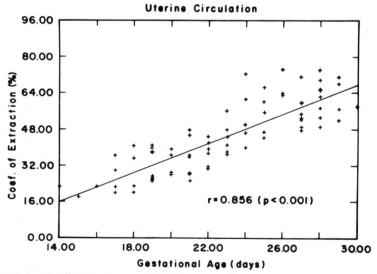

Figure 8-3:   Coefficient of oxygen utilization across the uterine circulation of rabbits in the last 15 days of pregnancy (37).

the pregnant uterus. Although the P_{O_2} of fetal blood may decrease in the entire course of gestation (reliable data about early fetal life are not yet available), it is important to emphasize that there is no evidence for a progressive deterioration in fetal oxygenation during the last month of ovine pregnancy. Daily sampling of fetal arterial blood in this period has demonstrated that under normal physiologic conditions, the P_{O_2} of fetal blood remains stable (34).

In relation to fetal weight and uterine oxygen demands, the rate of perfusion of the pregnant uterus is much higher in sheep than in rabbits and guinea pigs. For the rabbit the rate of uterine perfusion per millimole of oxygen consumed is considerably less than that for the body as a whole after approximately 20 days gestation (37). This is illustrated in Figure 8-4, which shows the ratio of the arteriovenous oxygen difference across the uterus to the arteriovenous oxygen difference across the lungs. A ratio of 1.0 would imply that in relation to oxygen demands the quantity of blood perfusing the uterus is the same as the quantity of blood perfusing the whole body. It is apparent that after approximately 20 days gestation the uterus of the rabbit is relatively underperfused compared to the whole

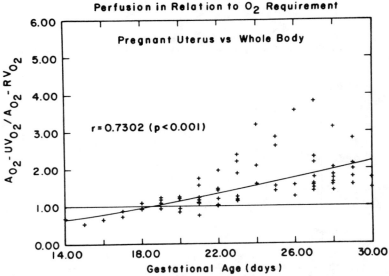

Figure 8-4: In pregnant rabbits the uterine : pulmonary arteriovenous oxygen difference ratio becomes greater than 1.0 after the 20th day of gestation. This observation indicates that, in relation to oxygen demands, the uterus in late pregnancy is relatively underperfused compared with the rest of the body (37).

Table 8-2

Comparison between Near Term Pregnant Sheep (130–140 Days Gestation), Rabbits (29 Days Gestation), and Guinea Pigs (58–67 Days Gestation)[a]

Blood flows	Sheep[b] $n = 7$	Rabbit[c] $n = 10$	Guinea pig[d] $n = 6$
Placental blood flow			
Per unit weight of fetus (ml/g/min)	0.26 ± 0.02	0.106 ± 0.008	0.114 ± 0.02
Per unit weight of placenta (ml/g/min)	2.8 ± 0.2	0.57 ± 0.05	1.56 ± 0.3
Fetal : maternal weight ratio	0.07	0.07 ± 0.01	0.25 ± 0.02
Uterine blood flow			
Percentage of cardiac output	15.7 ± 1.3	6.7 ± 0.7	12.8 ± 2.5
Mammary blood flow			
Per unit weight of organ (ml/g/min)	0.3 ± 0.03	0.37 ± 0.05	0.33 ± 0.07
Percentage of cardiac output	2.05 ± 0.3	5.1 ± 0.5	1.4 ± 0.3

[a] Values are given as mean ± SEM.
[b] Data from Rosenfeld (44).
[c] Data from Johnson et al. (23).
[d] Data from Myers et al. (38); data on guinea pig mammary blood flow from Peeters et al. (41).

body. Table 8-2 presents data we have obtained for the three species all studied under comparable steady-state, unstressed conditions. The two small mammals have placental blood flows per gram of fetus that are almost one-third the sheep value. This remarkable difference in the uterine perfusion rate required to supply the same fetal mass is related to differences in the effectiveness of transplacental exchange (as explained in Chapters 2 and 6). A placenta which is a venous equilibrator (e.g., the sheep placenta) requires a higher level of perfusion than a placenta which is a countercurrent exchanger in order to attain comparable levels of fetal oxygenation. The placental blood flows per gram of fetus presented in Table 8-2 are average values calculated for the purpose of interspecies comparison. It is important to note that within any given species, placental blood flows per gram of fetus have a relatively large coefficient of variation because placental flow and fetal weight are not proportional. For example, in the guinea pig, if one compares the largest and smallest fetuses within the same litter, they usually differ by approximately 30% in body weight. However, maternal placental blood flow is 95% greater in the larger fetus. Similarly, large placentas are "hyperperfused" per unit weight of placental tissue compared to the smaller placentas (38). In the guinea pig the low level of uterine perfusion required to grow 1 g of fetus is used to grow a very large fetal mass.

Newborn guinea pigs are quite mature and need very little nursing. By contrast, in rabbits the fetal : maternal weight ratio is kept small by a short gestation, and at term uterine blood flow is a smaller percentage of cardiac output than in sheep and guinea pigs. Since newborn rabbits are immature and require an abundant supply of milk, the mammary blood flow of rabbits near term is about as large as uterine blood flow, in sharp contrast to comparable data in sheep and guinea pigs (Table 8-2).

In pregnant women maternal cardiac output increases 30–40% in early gestation and then plateaus to approximately 6.8 liter/min (29). On the assumption that the human placenta has about the same low level of effectiveness as the ovine placenta, it is reasonable to estimate the normal level of uterine perfusion in late human pregnancy at approximately 1.0 liter/min or approximately 15% of maternal cardiac output.

PRESSURE–FLOW RELATIONSHIP

When the uterus is relaxed, blood flow through the placenta depends on the pressure difference between arterial and uterine venous blood. According to Greiss *et al.* (21), the flow–pressure relationship of the sheep placenta is quasilinear, being represented by a curve with gentle convexity toward the pressure axis and a 7.5 Torr intercept at zero flow. This evidence is important because it indicates that placental blood flow is not autoregulated, which means that a decrease in arterial pressure does not elicit a compensatory decrease in placental vascular resistance. Confirmatory evidence in other species is needed because of differences in placental structure. In sheep the main resistance to placental blood flow is contributed by the vasculature located within the placental cotyledons, whereas in hemochorial placentae the main resistance to placental blood flow is in the arterial tree supplying blood to the placenta (35, 36). These differences in the anatomic location of the resistance vessels suggest the possibility of a difference in regulation which should be explored by similar studies of flow-pressure relationships in hemochorial placentae.

When the pregnant uterus contracts, blood flow through the placenta no longer depends upon the arteriovenous pressure difference across the uterus but on the pressure difference between arterial blood and the uterine cavity. As the pressure within the uterine cavity (amniotic pressure) increases above abdominal pressure, it tends to collapse the placental vascular bed, thus creating a hindrance to the flow of blood. A negative correlation between amniotic pressure and placental blood flow has been

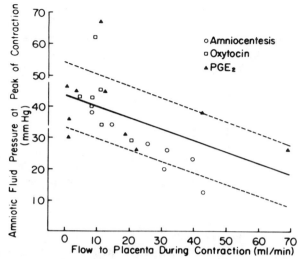

Figure 8-5: Inverse relationship of placental blood flow to intrauterine pressure in the rhesus monkey (39).

demonstrated by Novy *et al.* (39) in the rhesus monkey (Figure 8-5). Novy's work illustrates the decrease in placental blood flow which accompanies uterine contractions. Such observations help explain the fetal distress which accompanies tetanic contractions and prolonged labor in humans.

SHORT-TERM REGULATION

The increase of uteroplacental blood flow during pregnancy results primarily from the formation and growth of the placental vascular bed. The regulatory mechanisms that influence the development of the placental circulation are unknown. Most of the studies of uteroplacental circulation have focused on its short-term regulation.

Spontaneous variations of uterine blood flow have been observed in chronic animal preparations. In rhesus monkeys confined to restraining chairs, uterine artery blood flow and amniotic and arterial blood pressure had a circadian rhythm (22). The highest flows tended to occur during the night, whereas amniotic and arterial pressures peaked during the day. Among animals, differences between minimal and maximal flow rates ranged from 17 to 64% of the mean daily flow. In sheep daily fluctuations of uterine blood flow have also been observed, but with no apparent relation to the light-dark cycle. From the experimental viewpoint it is important to emphasize that in a placid, pregnant ewe kept in a quiet environment uterine blood flow can remain virtually constant for hours, thus permitting measurements of uterine oxygen and substrates uptakes under steady-state conditions.

Respiratory Gases

Given the importance of respiratory gases as regulators of cardiac output and its distribution, their effect on uteroplacental blood flow has been studied fairly extensively. All such studies indicate that the partial pressure of oxygen and CO_2 do not exert any appreciable direct control on the placental circulation of sheep. The following list summarizes the evidence.

1. Pregnant sheep were exposed to alternate periods of air breathing, inhalation of 15% oxygen in nitrogen, and inhalation of 100% oxygen (30). Neither hypoxia nor hyperoxia caused any physiologically significant change of uterine blood flow.

2. Uterine blood flow was measured before and after fetal death induced by the injection of a bolus of air into the fetal inferior vena cava. Fetal death was followed by an abrupt reduction of uterine oxygen uptake to 25% of its control value, causing a rise of uterine venous P_{O_2} and a decrease of uterine venous P_{CO_2}. Despite these changes which occurred within minutes, uterine blood flow remained constant for the first hour after fetal death (43).

3. Placental antipyrine clearance, which depends primarily upon placental perfusion, was not altered by maternal inhalation of 100% oxygen which exposed the placental vessels to very high maternal arterial oxygen tensions (4).

4. Variations of arterial P_{CO_2} within the 30–60 Torr range had no detectable effect on uteroplacental vascular resistance (53).

5. Finally, several investigators have observed that an acute temporary reduction of placental blood flow is not followed by a compensatory increase of flow over baseline (reactive hyperemia) (17, 28, 43).

Hormonal Regulation

In nonpregnant ovariectomized sheep the injection of either estradiol-17β (E_2) or estriol (E_1) causes a marked increase of blood flow to myometrium, endometrium, and caruncles, the sites on the uterine mucosa that interact with fetal trophoblast to form the placental cotyledons (46).

Blood flow begins to increase approximately 20 min after the injection, peaks at 100 min, and then declines slowly, returning to baseline over several hours. The infusion of cycloheximide, an inhibitor of protein synthesis, blocks the blood flow response to estrogens (25), indicating that this response, like most physiologic responses to steroid hormones, is mediated by the synthesis of specific proteins. Similarly, the injection of estrogens at 38 days of pregnancy causes also a large increase of blood flow to myometrium, endometrium, and placental cotyledons (49). However, the effect on placental blood flow decreases rapidly as pregnancy progresses. Late in pregnancy the injection of estrogens causes a vasodilation which is limited primarily to myometrium and endometrium. These data are summarized in Table 8-3.

Since placental cotyledons produce estrogens, it is conceivable that the arterioles of the placental cotyledons are already under intense, local estrogen stimulation under normal physiologic conditions. Thus, it would not be surprising to find that they are not responding to exogenous estrogens. It is possible, however, that other hormones influence the reactivity of placental vessels in late pregnancy and make these vessels refractory to estrogen action. Despite considerable effort directed at this question, the physiological role of estrogens in regulating placental blood flow remains unsettled.

Table 8-3

Effect of Estradiol-17β (E_2) on the Blood Flow to
Myometrium, Endometrium, Implantation Sites
(Caruncles), and Placenta in Sheep

	Before E_2 (ml of blood/min)	After E_2[a] (ml of blood/min)
Oophorectomized, nonpregnant[b]		
Myometrium	9.4 ± 1.8	102 ± 16
Endometrium	8.2 ± 2.4	95 ± 20
Caruncles	7.1 ± 2.1	70 ± 9
38 days pregnant[c]		
Myometrium	26.8	129.3
Endometrium	54.7	125.0
Caruncles	30.6	109.5
100–145 days pregnant[c]		
Myometrium	35.3 ± 5	122.7 ± 11
Endometrium	157.6 ± 23	314.9 ± 39
Placenta	906.2 ± 155	1138.0 ± 119

[a] Two hours after the intravenous injection of E_2 (1 μg/kg).

[b] Data from Rosenfeld et al. (46).

[c] Data from Rosenfeld et al. (48).

In sheep and rabbits uteroplacental blood flow can be markedly decreased by the infusion of catecholamines (1, 3, 7, 18, 26, 45, 48). The ovine uterine vasculature is quite sensitive to this constrictive effect. Doses of norepinephrine or epinephrine below the level necessary to produce a significant elevation of blood pressure cause a significant decrease in endometrial, myometrial, and placental blood flow (Table 8-4). This reduction in flow can be completely inhibited by phenoxybenzamine, an α blocker (18).

There are several indications that the renin-angiotensin system could be important in regulating the circulation of pregnant animals. Renin is synthesized by the human chorion (51). Furthermore, nephrectomized pregnant rabbits maintain detectable plasma levels of renin, the main source of which appears to be the uterus (13). In comparison to nonpregnant women, pregnant patients require the intravenous infusion of higher doses of angiotensin II to increase blood pressure 20 Torr above baseline (15). However, patients who develop eclampsia are as sensitive to the infusion of angiotensin II as nonpregnant patients. The relevance of this information to uterine blood flow maintenance and regulation is uncertain. In sheep, the intravenous infusion of angiotensin II, at a dose that produces a 20 Torr increase of pressure, has virtually no effect on the resistance of the uteroplacental vascular bed (11, 32).

In exploring the role of prostaglandins as regulators of uteroplacental blood flow, different investigators have obtained contradictory results. This confusion stems from the fact that the responsiveness of the uteroplacental vascular bed to prostaglandins and to prostaglandin synthesis inhibitors (e.g., Indomethacin) can vary according to the physiologic state

Table 8-4

Effects of Intravenous Infusion of Catecholamines
on Ovine Placental, Endometrial, and
Myometrial Blood Flow[a]

	Blood flow (% change)	
	Epinephrine[b]	Norepinephrine[c]
Placental cotyledons	-34.5 ± 4.6	-31.4 ± 4.6
Endometrium	-58.7 ± 5.3	-64.2 ± 3.0
Myometrium	-36.9 ± 6.4	-44.6 ± 4.0

[a] Values are given as means $\pm$ SE for doses of 0.29 ± 0.03 and 0.24 ± 0.04 μg/kg/min of epinephrine and norepinephrine, respectively.

[b] Data from Rosenfeld et al. (48).

[c] Data from Rosenfeld et al. (49).

of the preparation. For example, observations in sheep have demonstrated that indomethacin can cause a significant decrease of uteroplacental vascular resistance 2 days after surgery, but has no appreciable effect on the 7th day (8). A compounding difficulty arises because several prostaglandins stimulate uterine contractions. For example, the injection of prostaglandin E_2 (PGE_2) into the maternal circulation causes uterine contractions and a decrease of placental blood flow in both the rhesus monkey (39) and sheep (42). The infusion of PGE_2 in the fetal lamb, however, results in a small increase of maternal placental blood flow (31, 42). A likely explanation for such results is that the injection of PGE_2 into the mother causes both a relaxation of the placental resistance vessels and uterine contractions. The contractions increase the external pressure on the placental circulation and determine a decrease in placental blood flow despite the decrease in intrinsic vascular resistance. If PGE_2 is injected into the fetus, the vasodilatory effect becomes manifest because under these circumstances the PGE_2 concentration is much greater in the placenta than in the myometrium.

Neural Regulation

The uterus is endowed with adrenergic innervation, whereas cholinergic innervation is scarce or altogether absent. An interesting property of the uterine adrenergic nerves is their response to pregnancy (52). The nonpregnant guinea pig uterus has an abundance of fibers that can be stained by the catecholamine fluorescence technique. When the animal becomes pregnant the fluorescence begins to disappear, first from those parts of the uterus in close proximity to an implantation site and then from the whole organ. In the uterine regions remote from direct fetoplacental influence, the nerves remain capable of storing catecholamines, but in the perifetal regions this capacity is lost, suggesting fiber degeneration. The response of the uterine adrenergic nerves to pregnancy is probably mediated by progesterone, since progesterone treatment causes a decrease in the norepinephrine content of the nonpregnant uterus (6, 12). These histological observations suggest that the uterine vasculature should become insensitive to neuroadrenergic stimulation as pregnancy progresses, although concurrently it may become hypersensitive to circulatory catecholamines. Experiments in dogs agree with this suggestion (50), but similar studies in sheep have failed to demonstrate substantial differences between nonpregnant and pregnant animals in the sensitivity of uterine blood flow to neural stimulation and catecholamine injection.

The main uterine arteries of some species (human, guinea pig, dog, and pig) are endowed with a plexus of cholinergic fibers that do not extend into the uterus. A role for these fibers in dilating the uterine arteries during pregnancy has been suggested (5).

DEPENDENCE OF FETAL AND PLACENTAL METABOLISM ON UTEROPLACENTAL BLOOD FLOW

The dependence of placental metabolic exchange on uteroplacental blood flow was examined in preceding chapters, primarily in relation to models of transplacental diffusion (Chapter 2) and the respiratory function of the placenta (Chapter 6). Here we summarize and conclude the discussion of this topic.

It is perhaps obvious, but worthy of emphasis nevertheless, that in different experimental situations one can measure changes of placental blood flow that are numerically equal but radically different in their basic nature. To use an extreme example, placental blood flow could decrease to half of normal either because the perfusion rate of the whole placenta is decreased by half or because half of the placental circulation is not perfused while the other half is perfused at a normal rate. Therefore, the functional meaning of variations in placental blood flow needs to be analyzed in each experimental situation. This analysis requires a clear understanding of what happens to placental metabolic exchange when there is a variation in the rate of perfusion of the placental microcirculation with no effect on placental blood flow distribution or any other property of the placental exchanger (e.g., the dimensions of the placental membrane and the magnitude and distribution of umbilical blood flow). Under these conditions, changes in the rate of placental perfusion alter the placental uptake and exchange of metabolites by altering the mean concentrations of molecules to which the placental membrane is exposed. The largest effect of flow variations is on the mean concentration of substances that have a normally large extraction coefficient across the placental circulation. For example, consider substances x and y with normal extraction coefficients of 40% and 4%, respectively, across the placental circulation. One can estimate on the basis of the Fick principle that a decrease in placental blood flow to half its normal value will tend to decrease the placental venous concentration of x by two-thirds (from 0.6 to 0.2 of the arterial concentration), whereas it will tend to decrease the venous concentration of y by 4% only (from 0.96 to 0.92 of the arterial concentration). Quantitatively different effects on venous concentrations reflect different effects on the mean concentrations to which the placental membrane is exposed. Therefore, variations in placental blood flow which do not involve changes in other properties of the placental exchanger are selective in their effect. The importance of uteroplacental blood flow in determining the level of fetal oxygenation is related to the fact that the extraction coefficient of oxygen across the uterine circulation is relatively large, even under normal physiologic conditions. Conversely, the relatively small importance of uteroplacental blood flow in determining the level of fetal glycemia is related to the small uteroplacental extraction coefficient of glucose. This type of reasoning is generally applicable to problems of placental physiology.

An interesting application has been in evaluating the assumption that the placental clearance of dehydroisoandrosterone sulfate (DS) to estradiol in humans is an index of placental blood flow, in other words, that an abnormally low DS clearance indicates an abnormally low blood flow (14). Since in normal human gestations at term the clearance of DS to estradiol is only 20 ml/min, whereas placental blood flow is approximately 500 ml/min or higher, one can estimate that normally the magnitude of the extraction coefficient of DS across the human placental circulation is 4% (percent extraction coefficient = 100 × clearance/flow). This low coefficient indicates that the clearance of DS is not likely to be a sensitive index of changes in placental blood flow (9). In searching for a steroid with a placental metabolic clearance that is a reliable index of placental blood flow, it would be worthwhile to focus attention on steroids whose placental clearance is similar in magnitude to placental blood flow.

Several experiments have aimed at describing the physiologic effects of decreasing uteroplacental blood flow below normal. Despite the common aim there have been major differences in experimental design which must be carefully noted for a correct interpretation of the results.

In Chapters 2 and 6 we described experiments in which the uteroplacental blood flow of sheep was decreased by partial occlusion of the terminal aorta. The effect of this procedure on the placental transfer of ethanol and oxygen was explained in terms of the measured changes in uteroplacental blood flow and the venous equilibration model of transplacental exchange. Additional assumptions about changes in the properties of the placental exchanger, as for example, closure of placental capillaries with reduction in the placental diffusing capacity for oxygen, were not required to explain the data. Therefore, these experiments may represent a true instance of a decrease in the rate of perfusion of the whole placental membrane while other properties of the placental exchanger remain virtually constant. Further studies are required, however, to test the validity of this hypothesis.

In 1972 Creasy and collaborators (10) developed a method for studying the responses of the sheep fetus to a chronic reduction in uteroplacental blood flow. In this method the placental microcirculation is embolized by injecting microspheres into the uterine arteries. It is important to note that a reduction in the mass and surface of functional trophoblast must be one of the consequences of the embolization. This reduction affects indiscriminately the placental transfer of every metabolite and not just the transfer of molecules whose placental transport rate is sensitive to changes in the rate of placental perfusion. Therefore, the microembolization technique cannot establish the importance of placental perfusion relative to other aspects of placental function in controlling fetal growth.

Experiments in small mammals with hemochorial placentas have used the technique of ligating one end of the uterine arterial arcade to produce fetal growth retardation (16, 24, 27, 40, 54). Although in some instances this procedure may cause placental infarctions (27), Wigglesworth (54) showed that fetal growth retardation in rats can be produced without histologic evidence of infarction. Thus, it would seem that the first consequence of uterine arterial ligation is to decrease in some of the conceptuses the rate of perfusion of the whole placenta without reducing the surface of the placental membrane which is perfused by maternal blood. At the end of pregnancy, however, the growth retarded fetuses have, in addition to low levels of placental blood flows, abnormally small placentas (16). This is perhaps the most intriguing aspect of the experiments of arterial ligation in small mammals because it suggests that a chronic reduction in placental blood flow has an adverse effect on the growth and development of the trophoblast. The mechanisms by which this effect is mediated are unknown. Reductions in the mean oxygen pressure and mean nutrient concentrations in the placental circulation may alter trophoblastic growth and development directly or, more likely, via a complex sequence of events involving changes in fetal metabolism and hormonal milieu (24). In addition, we should not overlook the possibility that placental growth is inhibited by a decrease of pressure in the placental circulation.

REFERENCES

1. Anderson, S.G., Still, J.G. and Greiss, F.C. (1977). *Differential reactivity of the gravid uterine vasculatures: effects of norepinephrine.* American Journal of Obstetrics and Gynecology **129**, 293–298.
2. Barcroft, J. (1933). *The conditions of foetal respiration.* Lancet **2**, 1021–1024.
3. Barton, M.D., Killam, A.P. and Meschia, G. (1974). *Response of ovine uterine blood flow to epinephrine and norepinephrine.* Proceedings of the Society for Experimental Biology and Medicine **145**, 996–1003.
4. Battaglia, F.C., Meschia, G., Makowski, E.L. and Bowes, W. (1968). *The effect of*

maternal oxygen inhalation upon fetal oxygenation. Journal of Clinical Investigation **47**, 548–555.

5. Bell, C. (1968). *Dual vasoconstrictor and vasodilator innervation of the uterine arterial supply in the guinea pig.* Circulation Research **23**, 279–289.

6. Bell, C. and Malcolm, S.J. (1978). *Observations on the loss of catecholamine fluorescence from intrauterine adrenergic nerves during pregnancy in the guinea pig.* Journal of Reproduction and Fertility **53**, 51–58.

7. Carter, A.M. and Olin, T. (1972). *Effect of adrenergic stimulation and blockade on the uteroplacental circulation and uterine activity in the rabbit.* Journal of Reproduction and Fertility **29**, 251–260.

8. Clark, K.E., Stys, S.J., Austin, J.E. and Golter, M. (1980). *Post surgical effects of indomethacin on uterine blood flow.* Society for Gynecologic Investigation, 27th Annual meeting, Denver, p 37.

9. Clewell, W. and Meschia, G. (1976). *Relationship of the metabolic clearance rate of dehydroisoandrosterone sulfate to placental blood flow: A mathematical model.* American Journal of Obstetrics and Gynecology **125**, 507–508.

10. Creasy, R.K., Barrett, C.T., DeSwiet, M., Kahanpaa, K.V. and Rudolph, A.M. (1972). *Experimental intrauterine growth retardation in the sheep.* American Journal of Obstetrics and Gynecology **112**, 566–573.

11. Edelstone, D.I., Botti, J.J., Mueller-Heubach, E. and Caritis, S.N. (1978). *Response of the circulation of pregnant sheep to angiotensin and norepinephrine before and after dexamethasone.* American Journal of Obstetrics and Gynecology **130**, 689–792.

12. Falck, B., Owman, C., Rosengren, E. and Sjoberg, N.-O. (1969). *Reduction by progesterone of the estrogen-induced increase in transmitter level of the short adrenergic neurons innervating the uterus.* Endocrinology **84**, 958–959.

13. Ferris, T.F., Stein, J.H. and Kauffman, J. (1972). *Uterine blood flow and uterine renin secretion.* Journal of Clinical Investigation **51**, 2827–2833.

14. Gant, N.F., Hutchison, H.T., Siiteri, P.K. and MacDonald, P.C. (1971). *Study of the metabolic clearance rate of dehydroisoandrosterone sulfate in pregnancy.* American Journal of Obstetrics and Gynecology **111**, 556–563.

15. Gant, N.F., Daley, G.L., Chand, S., Whalley, P.J. and MacDonald, P.C. (1973). *A study of angiotensin II pressor response throughout primigravid pregnancy.* Journal of Clinical Investigation **52**, 2682–2689.

16. Gilbert, M. and Leturque, A. (1982). *Fetal weight and its relationship to placental blood flow and placental weight in experimental intrauterine growth retardation.* Journal of Developmental Physiology **4**, 237–246.

17. Greiss, F.C. Jr. (1966). *Pressure–flow relationship in the gravid uterine vascular bed.* American Journal of Obstetrics and Gynecology **96**, 41–46.

18. Greiss, F.C. Jr. (1972). *Differential reactivity of the myoendometrial and placental vasculatures: adrenergic responses.* American Journal of Obstetrics and Gynecology **112**, 20–30.

19. Greiss, F.C. Jr. and Anderson, S.G. (1969). *Uterine vascular changes during the ovarian cycle.* American Journal of Obstetrics and Gynecology **103**, 629–640.

20. Greiss, F.C. Jr. and Anderson, S.B. (1970). *Uterine blood flow during early ovine pregnancy.* American Journal of Obstetrics and Gynecology **106**, 30–38.

21. Greiss, F.C. Jr., Anderson, S.G. and Still, J.G. (1976). *Uterine pressure–flow relationships during early gestation.* American Journal of Obstetrics and Gynecology **126**, 799–808.

22. Harbert, G.M. Jr. (1977). *Biorhythms of the pregnant uterus (Macaca mulatta).* American Journal of Obstetrics and Gynecology **129**, 401–408.

23. Johnson, R.L., Gilbert, M., Meschia, G. and Battaglia, F.C. (1985). *Cardiac output distribution and uteroplacental blood flow in the pregnant rabbit: A comparative study.* American Journal of Obstetrics and Gynecology **151**, 682–689.

24. Jones, C.T., Lafeber, H.N. and Roebuck, M.M. (1984). *Studies on the growth of the fetal guinea pig. Changes in plasma hormone concentration during normal and abnormal growth.* Journal of Developmental Physiology **6**, 461–472.

25. Killam, A.P., Rosenfeld, C.R., Battaglia, F.C., Makowski, E.L. and Meschia, G. (1973). *Effect of estrogens on the uterine blood flow of oophorectomized ewes.* American Journal of Obstetrics and Gynecology **115**, 1045–1052.

26. Ladner, C., Brinkman, C.R. III, Weston, P. and Assali, N.S. (1970). *Dynamics of uterine circulation in pregnant and nonpregnant sheep.* American Journal of Physiology **218**, 257–263.

27. Lafeber, H.N., Rolph, T.P. and Jones, C.T. (1984). *Studies on the growth of the fetal guinea pig. The effects of ligation of the uterine artery on organ growth and development.* Journal of Developmental Physiology **6**, 441–459.

28. Lees, M.H., Hill, J.D., Ochsner, A.J. III, Thomas, C.L. and Novy, M.J. (1971). *Maternal placental and myometrial blood flow of the rhesus monkey during uterine contractions.* American Journal of Obstetrics and Gynecology **110**, 68–81.

29. Lees, M.M., Taylor, S.H., Scott, D.B. and Kerr, M.G. (1967). *A study of cardiac output at rest throughout pregnancy.* Journal of Obstetrics and Gynaecology of the British Commonwealth **74**, 319–328.

30. Makowski, E.L., Hertz, R.H. and Meschia, G. (1973). *Effects of acute maternal hypoxia and hyperoxia on the blood flow to the pregnant uterus.* American Journal of Obstetrics and Gynecology **115**, 624–631.

31. McLaughlin, M., Brennan, S.C. and Chez, R.A. (1978). *Vasoconstrictive effects of prostaglandins in sheep placental circulations.* American Journal of Obstetrics and Gynecology **130**, 408–413.

32. McLaughlin, M.K., Brennan, S.C. and Chez, R.A. (1978). *Effects of indomethacin on sheep uteroplacental circulations and sensitivity to angiotensin II.* American Journal of Obstetrics and Gynecology **132**, 430–435.

33. Meschia, G. (1984). *Circulation to female reproductive organs. In* "Handbook of Physiology. The Cardiovascular System," (J.T. Shepherd and F.M. Abboud, eds.), Volume III, pp 241–269, American Physiological Society, Bethesda, Maryland.

34. Meschia, G., Makowski, E.L. and Battaglia, F.C. (1970). *The use of indwelling catheters in the uterine and umbilical veins of sheep for a description of fetal acid–base balance and oxygenation.* Yale Journal of Biology and Medicine **42**, 154–165.

35. Moll, W. and Kunzel, W. (1973). *The blood pressure in arteries entering the placentae of guinea pigs, rats, rabbits and sheep.* Pfluegers Archives **338**, 125–131.

36. Moll, W., Kunzel, W., Stolte, L.A.M., Kleinhout, J., Dejong, P.A. and Veth, A.F.L. (1974). *The blood pressure in the decidual part of the uteroplacental arteries (spiral arteries) of the rhesus monkey.* Pfluegers Archives **346**, 291–297.

37. Murray, R.D., Jones, R.O., Johnson, R.L., Meschia, G. and Battaglia, F.C. (1985). *Uterine and whole body oxygen extractions in the pregnant rabbit under chronic steady-state conditions.* American Journal of Obstetrics and Gynecology **152**, 709–715.

38. Myers, S., Sparks, J.W., Makowski, E.L., Meschia, G. and Battaglia, F.C. (1982). *The relationship between placental blood flow and placental and fetal size in guinea pig.* American Journal of Physiology **243**, H404–H409.

39. Novy, M.J., Thomas, C.L. and Lees, M.H. (1975). *Uterine contractility and regional blood flow responses to oxytocin and prostaglandin E_2 in pregnant rhesus monkeys.* American Journal of Obstetrics and Gynecology **122**, 419–433.

40. Oh, W., D'Amodio, M.D., Yap, L.L. and Hohenauer, L. (1970). *Carbohydrate metabolism in experimental intrauterine growth retardation in rats*. American Journal of Obstetrics and Gynecology **108**, 415–421.

41. Peeters, L.L.H., Grutters, G. and Martin, C.B. (1980). *Distribution of cardiac output in the unstressed pregnant guinea pig*. American Journal of Obstetrics and Gynecology **138**, 1177–1184.

42. Rankin, J.H.G. and Phernetton, T.M. (1976). *Effect of prostaglandin E_2 on ovine maternal placental blood flow*. American Journal of Physiology **231**, 754–759.

43. Raye, J.R., Killam, A.P., Battaglia, F.C., Makowski, E.L. and Meschia. G. (1971). *Uterine blood flow and O_2 consumption following fetal death in sheep*. American Journal of Obstetrics and Gynecology **111**, 917–924.

44. Rosenfeld, C.R. (1977). *Distribution of cardiac output in ovine pregnancy*. American Journal of Physiology **232**, H231–H235.

45. Rosenfeld, C.R. and West, J. (1977). *Circulatory response to systemic infusion of norepinephrine in the pregnant ewe*. American Journal of Obstetrics and Gynecology **127**, 376–383.

46. Rosenfeld, C.R., Killam, A.P., Battaglia, F.C., Makowski, E.L. and Meschia, G. (1973). *Effect of estradiol-17β on the magnitude and distribution of uterine blood flow in nonpregnant, oophorectomized ewes*. Pediatric Research **7**, 139–148.

47. Rosenfeld, C.R., Morriss, F.H. Jr., Makowski, E.L., Meschia, G. and Battaglia, F.C. (1974). *Circulatory changes in the reproductive tissues of ewes during pregnancy*. Gynecological Investigation **5**, 252–268.

48. Rosenfeld, C.R., Barton, M.D. and Meschia, G. (1976). *Effects of epinephrine on distribution of blood flow in the pregnant ewe*. American Journal of Obstetrics and Gynecology **124**, 156–163.

49. Rosenfeld, C.R., Morriss, F.H. Jr., Battaglia, F.C., Makowski, E.L. and Meschia, G. (1976). *Effect of estradiol-17β on blood flow to reproduction and nonreproductive tissues in pregnant ewes*. American Journal of Obstetrics and Gynecology **124**, 618–629.

50. Ryan, M.J., Clark, K.E. and Brody, M.J. (1974). *Neurogenic and mechanical control of canine uterine vascular resistance*. American Journal of Physiology **227**, 547–555.

51. Symonds, E.M., Stanley, M.A. and Skinner, S.L. (1968). *Production of renin by* in vitro *cultures of human chorion and uterine muscle*. Nature London **217**, 1152–1153.

52. Thorbert, G., Alm, P., Owman, C., Sjoberg, N.-O. and Sporrong, B. (1978). *Regional changes in structural and functional integrity of myometrial adrenergic nerves in pregnant guinea-pig, and their relationship to the localization of the conceptus*. Acta Physiology Scandanavia **103**, 120–131.

53. Walker, A.M., Oakes, G.K., Ehrenkranz, R., McLaughlin, M. and Chez, R.A. (1976). *Effects of hypercapnia on uterine and umbilical circulations in conscious pregnant sheep*. Journal of Applied Physiology **41**, 727–733.

54. Wigglesworth, J.C. (1964). *Experimental growth retardation in the foetal rat*. Journal of Pathology and Bacteriology **88**, 1–13.

9

Fetal Water Balance

GENERAL CONSIDERATIONS

During its growth the fetus accumulates water in both the intra- and extracellular spaces (see Chapter 1). In addition, the fluids surrounding the fetus increase in volume for most of gestation. This may be confined to the amniotic fluid, as in humans, or include the allantoic as well as amniotic fluids, as in ungulates. Water accumulation is particularly striking in early pregnancy when the fetus represents a relatively small mass of tissue with a high water concentration, surrounded by a much larger volume of fluid. In order for the placenta to transfer a net quantity of water sufficient to account for this accumulation, there must be a driving force from maternal to fetal plasma.

Early attempts to identify the driving force for water were focused on three possible mechanisms: (a) an osmotic pressure gradient across the placenta such that the osmolality of fetal fluids were higher than maternal, (b) a colloidal osmotic pressure higher in the fetal than the maternal plasma, or (c) a pressure difference between the maternal and fetal placental microcirculations. There is an interesting history to the studies which were directed at determining how water accumulation occurs on the fetal side of the placenta. Early studies suggested that in some species, for example the sheep, there is a rather large osmotic gradient across the placenta with the fetus considerably hypertonic with respect to the maternal plasma (23). These early studies were carried out on material obtained from slaughterhouses where the fetal blood was sampled after the mother and fetus were killed. However, when investigators were first able to carry out studies under chronic steady-state conditions, the total osmotic pressures measured in fetal and maternal plasmas were virtually identical. In fact, the fetal plasma was slightly hypotonic with respect to the maternal plasma (Figure 9-1) (22). In order to understand the earlier reports of a large osmotic pressure difference between fetus and mother, we carried out studies on the effect of severe hypoxia on plasma osmolality (2). Such studies demonstrated that hypoxia causes a marked rise in plasma total osmotic pressure (Figure 9-2). The increase in plasma total osmotic pressure is due to an increase in intracellular osmolality with hypoxia, but the components which increase in the plasma depend upon the metabolic response to hypoxia. When there is no hyperglycemia associated with hypoxia, the shift of water from extra- to intracellular space leads to an increase in plasma sodium and chloride concentrations. This shift is minimized when there is a concomitant hyperglycemia. The osmotic pressure gradient between fetal and maternal plasmas described in earlier studies is now quite understandable. Clearly, differences in total osmotic pressure between maternal and fetal plasma will not explain the net accumulation of water on the fetal side of the placenta.

This is also true for differences in colloidal osmotic pressure. The colloidal osmotic pressure of fetal plasma is considerably less than that of

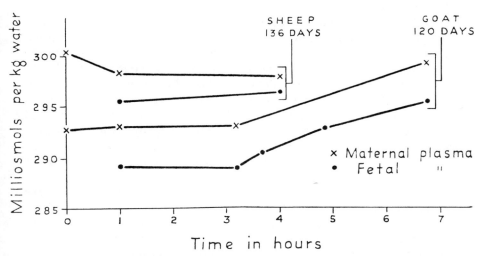

Figure 9-1:   The relationship between the total osmotic pressures of the maternal and fetal blood in a sheep and a goat when sampled twice or more in the course of the experiment (22).

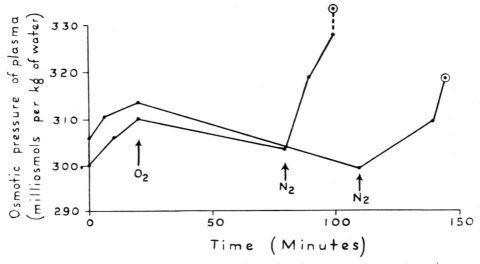

Figure 9-2: At time zero the two rabbits started to breathe nitrogen. Twenty minutes later they were allowed to breathe air again. At 80 and 110 min, respectively, they started once again to breathe nitrogen. The points enclosed in a circle indicate that the samples were taken immediately after the heart had ceased beating (2).

maternal plasma. The reasons for this vary among species. Figure 9-3 (11) illustrates the colloidal osmotic pressure in human fetal and maternal plasmas. The lower colloidal osmotic pressure in the human fetus reflects primarily a lower protein concentration (4). The colloidal osmotic pressure per gram of protein in maternal and fetal plasma are similar but not identical because the IGM class of immune globulins is not transferred across the human placenta. In the fetal sheep, where no immune globulins are transferred across the placenta and where the plasma protein concentration is low (approximately 4 to 5 g/dl at term), the plasma colloidal osmotic pressure is not much lower than in the human fetus because of the presence of large quantities of proteins with a relatively low molecular weight. One of these proteins, fetuin, is characteristic of fetal life (21). Note that values reported for plasma colloidal osmotic pressure are a function of the pore size of the membrane used in the pressure measurement. The larger the pore size of the membrane used, the lower the colloidal osmotic pressure. This is important not only in relation to placenta water transfer but also in considering fluid shifts between the intravascular and interstitial fluid compartments within the fetus. It would be necessary to have detailed information on the permeability characteristics of the endothelial membrane in the various organs to be able to interpret

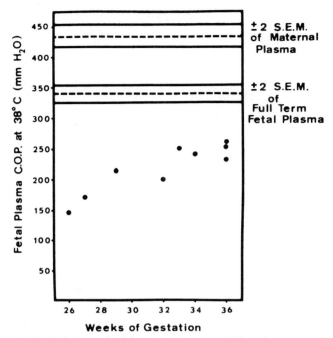

Figure 9-3: Fetal plasma colloidal osmotic pressure (COP) in humans versus gestational age. The maternal and fetal plasma colloidal osmotic pressures at term ± 2 SEM are also shown for comparison (11).

the physiological meaning of a given colloidal osmotic pressure measurement. Since this information is not available for fetuses, measurements of colloidal osmotic pressure provide only a rough guideline of some of the forces controlling fluid shifts between fetal water compartments.

The measurements of total and colloidal osmotic pressure make it clear that transplacental gradients for either of these pressures could not account for a net water transfer to the fetus. However, this knowledge does not invalidate the hypothesis that the sum of the osmotic forces exerted by each plasma solute across the placental membrane favors the transport of water from mother to fetus. To test this hypothesis, it would be necessary to determine the placental reflection coefficients of solutes in maternal and fetal plasma. This is a much more difficult task than measuring osmolarities and colloidal osmotic pressures. Permeability constants of different solutes have been measured by Boyd *et al.* (5, 6) for the sheep placenta under *in vivo* steady-state conditions. Table 9-1 from one of their reports presents their data. The relative impermeability of the sheep pla-

Table 9-1

Some Mean Permeability Constants (K):
Sheep Placenta Near Term[a,b]

Permeant	Molecular weight	$K \pm$ SEM (ml/min)	n
Urea	60	61 ± 6	11
Erythritol	122	1.8 ± 0.2	12
Mannitol	182	0.17 ± 0.04	6
Cr EDTA	387	0.007	2
α-Methylglucoside	194	-0.02 ± 0.05	3
3-O-Methylglucose	194	62 ± 7	11

[a] Permeability values are uncorrected for blood flow limitation; n is number of injections of each isotope, each injection being followed by 5–10 individual measurements of K.

[b] From Boyd et al. (6).

centa to water soluble polar molecules is apparent and suggests that these compounds may have reflection coefficients approaching 1.0. Faber and Thornburg (12) attempted to estimate the placental reflection coefficients of sodium and chloride. Their values are reasonable (0.83 and 0.79, respectively) given the low placental permeability to these ions. For example, Boyd et al. (6) reported very small unidirectional sodium fluxes in both directions for the sheep placenta. These fluxes, not surprisingly, were a function of fetal weight, but at all weights they were extremely low when compared to that of urea or of substances with flow-limited clearance. Nevertheless, there are many pitfalls in attempting to estimate placental reflection coefficients, and without knowledge of these coefficients the osmotic effect of transplacental concentration gradients cannot be precisely defined. The issue of whether a pressure difference between the maternal and fetal placental microcirculations can be a significant factor in transferring water across the placenta is unsettled. Faber and Thornburg (12) have proposed a theory in which pressure differences across the placenta play a crucial role in fetal water balance and circulatory homeostasis. They have postulated, for example, that an increase of fetal placental capillary pressure above its steady-state value would lead to a loss of fetal fluids across the placenta into the maternal circulation, producing a reduction in fetal blood volume and fetal heart filling pressure. This in turn would decrease both fetal cardiac output and fetal placental blood flow and capillary pressure. These compensatory changes would lead to the reestablishment of a new steady state. We have seen, however, that the epithelium of the sheep placental membrane is relatively impermeable to small molecules. This creates a condition in which nearly every solute concentration difference across the epithelium is capable of exerting an osmotic force. At body temperature and for solutes with a reflection coefficient of 1.0, small concentration differences represent a large osmotic force (1 mmol/kg of water concentration difference exerts an osmotic pressure of 19 Torr). Therefore, it is uncertain whether physiologic pressure differences of a few torr between maternal and fetal blood in the placenta can represent anything more than a small component of the set of forces moving water and solutes across the placental barrier.

Another major problem in attempting to study what governs water transfer across the placenta to the fetus to accommodate for fetal growth is that the quantities of water required are very small in relationship to gestation length. For example, Faber and Thornburg (12) have estimated that the water required for fetal growth in the late gestation fetal lamb would only be equal to 17.4 μl/kg/min; this flux would require an osmotic gradient too small for detection. The discussion in Chapter 3 regarding the limitations of an application of the Fick principle to measurements of the net transfer of compounds across the placenta applies just as stringently to this area of water and mineral transport. The quantities transferred of substances such as sodium, potassium, and calcium, which are not metabolized but accumulate with growth, are so small when delivered over the entire period of gestation as well as relative to blood flow in the fetal and maternal circulations that it is impossible to arrive at estimates of net transfer from measurements of arteriovenous differences. Similarly, relatively large net movements of water between placenta and fetus cannot be detected by measuring differences in water content between umbilical arterial and venous blood.

While absolute values for placental water clearance vary among species, in all species the placental permeability to water molecules is very great. Thus, when osmotic gradients are created across the placenta experimentally by infusions of hypertonic saline, mannitol, etc., a net water transfer quickly reestablishes osmotic equilibrium. When the hypertonic solution is infused into the mother, the net transfer of water is from the fetal to the maternal circulation leading to fetal dehydration. This was first demonstrated in pregnant rabbits (Figure 9-4) (8) and later in pregnant rhesus monkeys and their fetuses (8).

There are clinical implications to these observations that osmotic gradients tend to equilibrate fairly rapidly across the placenta. There have been numerous reports of neonatal hyponatremia and hypotonicity occurring in infants whose mothers had developed hyponatremia secondary to water intoxication. The usual situation in which this can occur is one in which the pregnant woman is receiving intravenous glucose solutions for the

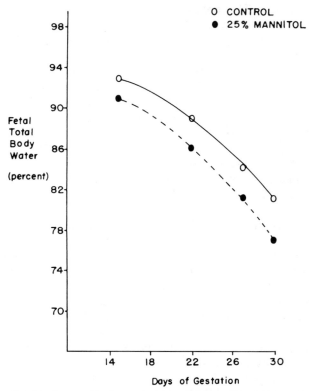

Figure 9-4: Total body water in the normal fetus decreased from 93% at the 15th day of gestation to 81% near term. The maternal infusion of 25% mannitol resulted in a mean decrease of 3% in the water content of the fetus. This net transfer of water from fetus to mother was highly significant throughout gestation (7).

administration of some drug such as oxytocin or tocolytics, and the quantity of fluid is overlooked as attention is focused upon titration of the biological effect of the drug. As the maternal sodium concentration falls from dilution by the infusate, water moves from the maternal to the fetal circulation and, to a lesser extent, sodium ions move in the opposite direction, leading to fetal hyponatremia and osmotic equilibration across the placenta (3).

The issue of measuring the net placental transfer of water from mother to fetus has been addressed by Lumbers *et al.* (19). They blocked fetal swallowing and directly determined lung and urine flow rates in the fetal lamb. They assumed that under these experimental conditions the net amount of water gained by the fetus via the placenta is equal to the amount of water lost via the urinary and pulmonary output, plus the water deposited in the growing fetal tissues minus the water produced by fetal oxidative metabolism. The combined flux thus estimated was 0.4 ± 0.09 ml/kg/min. The fetal urinary flow rates they reported represented approximately 70% of this flux, and the lung fluid flow rate represented approximately 20%. The water accumulating in the fetus as a function of growth was estimated at 2.3×10^{-2} ml/kg/min or 6% of the transplacental flux. Clearly, however, the value of 0.4 ml/kg/min does not represent normal net transplacental water flux since fetal swallowing and water reabsorption through the amniotic and allantoic membranes would return to the fetus most of the fluids excreted via the lung and kidney.

In Chapter 1 we described the growth curve of the fetal lamb as well as its changing water content. For the reasons described in that chapter, the net accumulation of water in the fetus will vary at different stages of development. However, if one accepts the value of 2.3×10^{-2} ml/kg/min as reasonable for the latter 20% of gestation, then we can compare the water generated by metabolism with that required for accumulation in new tissues as growth.

For glucose the calculations yield approximately 0.15 g of water/kcal and for an average protein containing 52% carbon, 7% hydrogen, 23% oxygen, and 17% nitrogen, the combustion of 100 g would yield 41.4 g of water, or 0.09 g of water/kcal. The data reviewed in Chapters 3 and 4 suggest that in the fetal lamb a mixture of approximately 70% carbohydrate and 30% amino acids may be catabolized. Thus, a figure of $(0.7)(0.15) + (0.3)(0.09) = 0.13$ g of water/kcal would be reasonable for the estimation of water oxidation. The metabolic rate of the term fetal lamb is approximately 3.5×10^{-2} kcal/kg/min. Therefore, the water generated by metabolism equals $(3.5 \times 10^{-2})(0.13) = 4.55 \times 10^{-3}$ g/kg/min, which would represent approximately 20% of the water accretion in the fetus.

INTRAAMNIOTIC FLUID DYNAMICS

Figure 9-5 presents a diagram of the interorgan relationships that determine amniotic fluid volume in fetuses with no allantoic sac. Unidirectional arrows are shown for the kidney and lung into amniotic fluid since these organs contribute a net flow of fluid into the amniotic cavity. Conversely, there is a net absorption of amniotic fluid through the fetal gastrointestinal tract. There are no quantitative data about a net water flow through the amniotic membrane between amnion and the fetal or maternal circulation, although a bidirectional exchange of water molecules clearly occurs (15).

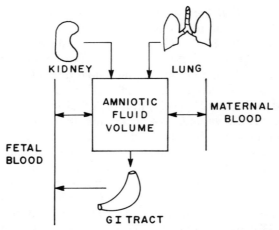

Figure 9-5: Diagram of water fluxes in and out of the amniotic fluid. The diagram excludes an appreciable allantoic cavity.

The absolute values for the net flow would be quite different at different stages of gestation and certainly among different species. In those species that maintain an allantoic sac, there is a varying contribution of fetal urine to both the allantoic and amniotic cavities. Changes in ovine amniotic and allantoic volumes and in fetal water content are presented in Figure 9-6

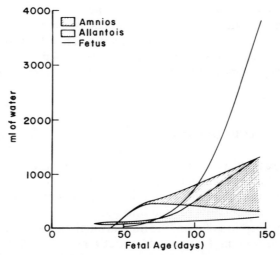

Figure 9-6: The accumulation of water in the fetal lamb and in the amniotic and allantoic cavities during gestation. From data by Cloete (10).

(10). The osmolality of amniotic fluid decreases with increasing gestational age, which reflects the increasing contribution of fetal urine to amniotic fluid composition (16). Fetal urine production in humans and sheep has been reasonably well studied and is characterized by a high flow rate and low osmolality. Early observations in our laboratory were made upon fetal lambs whose bladders were catheterized chronically via the urachus. Figure 9-7 presents these data and illustrates the fetal renal response to stress (13). The urine is hypertonic immediately after surgery and stabilizes after 3–5 days at a high flow rate and low osmolality. Just

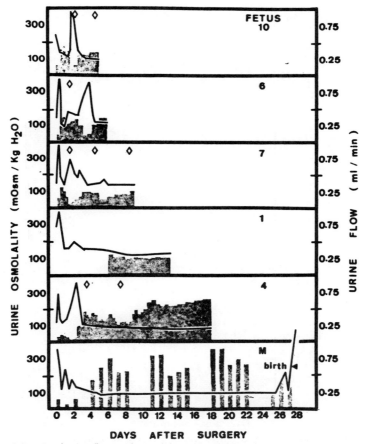

Figure 9-7: Fetal urine flow and osmolality. Osmolalities are represented by the solid line, and urine flows and sampling intervals are shown by the bar graphs. The diamonds indicate the times of clearance studies (13). Reproduced from *The Journal of Clinical Investigation,* 1972, **51,** 149–156, by copyright permission of The American Society for Clinical Investigation.

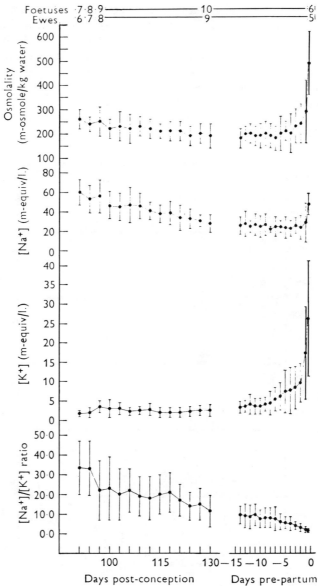

Figure 9-8: The mean ± SD over 3-day intervals for osmolality, [Na+], [K+], and [Na+] : [K+] ratio of fetal urine from a maximum of ten fetuses in nine ewes between 91 and 120 days gestational age, and their daily mean ± SD during the last 14 days before birth (20).

before delivery the urine again becomes hypertonic, perhaps reflecting vasopressin release by the fetus in response to the stress induced by parturition. In later studies Mellor and Slater (20) confirmed this pattern in more detailed studies. Figure 9-8 presents their data, again illustrating the low osmolality of fetal urine and the increase prior to delivery. It is interesting that estimates of fetal urine production by the human fetus gave similar values (approximately 0.1–0.2 ml/kg/min) as those found in the fetal lamb (Figure 9-9) (26).

FETAL LUNG FLUID

Fetal lung fluid electrolyte composition is shown in Table 9-2 (25). Fetal lung fluid is fairly close to plasma in its osmolality (1). Given this observation and the hypotonicity of fetal urine, it seems reasonable to interpret the decreasing osmolality of amniotic fluid during gestation as a reflection of the increasing contribution of fetal urine to its production. The regulation of fetal lung fluid has received a great deal of attention because of its significance in neonatal respiratory disease (17). Jost and Policard (18) first described the fact that fluid was produced in the fetal lungs and

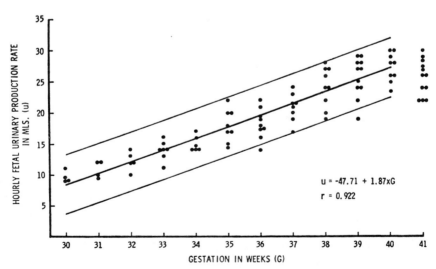

Figure 9-9: Relationship between human fetal urine production rate and the menstrual age of the fetus from 30 to 41 weeks in normal pregnancy (92 cases) (26).

Table 9-2

Composition of Lung Liquid, Lung Lymph, and Plasma
in Mature Fetal Lambs (in mEq/kg H_2O)[a,b]

Composition	Lung liquid[c]	Lung lymph[c]	Plasma[c]	$R_{p/LL}$[d]	$R_{p/uf}$[e]	Amniotic liquid
Na^+	150 ± 1.3	147 ± 0.6	150 ± 0.7	1.03	1.05	113 ± 6.5
K^+	6.3 ± 0.7	4.8 ± 0.5	4.8 ± 0.2	0.72	1.04	7.6 ± 0.8
Cl^-	157 ± 4.1	107 ± 0.9	107 ± 0.9	0.68	0.96	87 ± 5.0
HCO_3^-	2.8 ± 0.3	25 ± 0.8	24 ± 1.2	8.61	0.96	19 ± 3.0
Phosphates as P	0.02	—	2.3 ± 0.17	—	—	3.2
Ca^{2+}	0.22 ± 0.015[f]	—	0.62 ± 0.051[f]	2.82	1.53[g]	—
pH	6.27 ± 0.05	7.31 ± 0.02	7.34 ± 0.04	0.09	—	7.02 ± 0.9
Urea	7.9 ± 2.7	—	8.2 ± 1.4	—	—	10.5 ± 2.4
P_{CO_2} (mmHg)	40 ± 3	—	43 ± 4	—	—	54 ± 7
Protein osmotic pressure (mmHg)	1.0	17.4 ± 1.5	28.2 ± 1.2	—	—	1.0
(Protein) (g/dl)	0.027 ± 0.002	3.27 ± 0.41	4.09 ± 0.26	—	—	0.10 ± 0.01
Osmolality (mOsmol/kg H_2O)	294 ± 2	—	291 ± 2	—	—	265 ± 2

[a] Values are given as mean ± SE.

[b] From Strang (25).

[c] The water content of the liquids is as follows: plasma = 956 g/liter; lymph = 960 g/liter; lung liquid = 990 g/liter.

[d] $R_{p/LL}$ is plasma/lung liquid; for pH the ratio refers to H^+.

[e] $R_{p/uf}$ is plasma/ultrafiltrate, from Davson (10a).

[f] Measured with Ca^{2+} selective electrode.

[g] Assumes ionized Ca^{2+} is 0.67 of total.

delivered into amniotic fluid rather than the converse. Since then research has centered around how the fluid is produced, what tissues in the lung represent the sites of production, and what regulates its absorption or secretion. Lung fluid flow rate estimates have varied from approximately 0.04 to 0.08 ml/kg/min depending upon the techniques used for its measurement. For reviews of this area and of the factors controlling lung fluid reabsorption during parturition, we recommend reviews by Olver (24) and Strang (25).

Fetal lung fluid has also been studied intensively for its surfactant properties, again, stimulated by the clinical relevance to hyaline membrane disease, a frequent cause of severe respiratory distress in prematurely

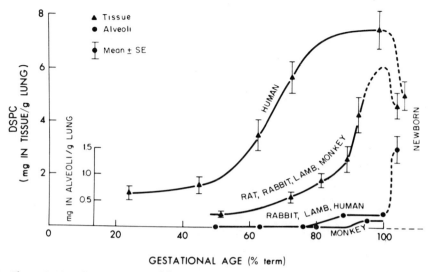

Figure 9-10:   Concentrations of disaturated phosphatidylcholine (DSPC) in lung tissue and alveoli plotted against relative gestational age for rats, rabbits, lambs, monkeys and humans. Values are averaged over intervals of 10 to 20% of gestation according to local density of data. The number of data points on which the curves are based are tissue, 20 (human); tissue, 34 (rat 7, rabbit 6, lamb 11, monkey 10); alveoli, 57 (rabbit 9, lamb 28, human 20); and alveoli, 40 (monkey). Reprinted from Ref. 9 by permission of Marcel Dekker, Inc.

born infants. The composition of surfactant has been fairly well described. Clements and Tooley (9) reviewed the choices of substances whose concentrations could be followed in fetal lung fluid as a reflection of surfactant concentration. Figure 9-10 from their report illustrates the changes in phosphatidycholine in lung tissue and its abrupt increase in alveoli for several species (9). Other phospholipids also show a characteristic developmental pattern during gestation, the pattern varying in different species. Figure 9-11 taken from the report of Hallman *et al.* (14) illustrates the amniotic fluid changes for two phospholipids, phophatidylinositol and phosphatidylglycerol, which arise from the lung fluid of human fetuses. Based on these changes, a variety of amniotic fluid tests have been developed that can be used clinically to predict in advance of delivery that the fetal lung is mature, at least in its surfactant properties. However, with improvements in ultrasonic evaluation of the fetus and other biophysical tests, amniotic fluid tests of pulmonary maturity are not used as extensively as they were some years ago.

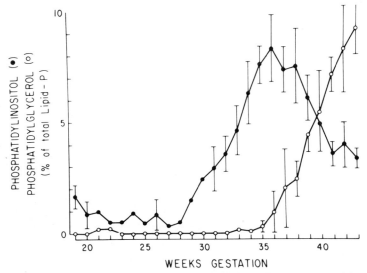

Figure 9-11: Changes in the content of phosphatidylglycerol and phosphatidylinositol in amniotic fluid during late gestation. The percentage of phosphatidylinositol and phosphatidylglycerol as measured by phosphate content in amniotic fluid samples from normal pregnancies is expressed versus gestational age (values are mean ± SD) (14).

REFERENCES

1. Adamson, T.M., Boyd, R.D.H., Platt, H.S. and Strang, L.B. (1969). *Composition of alveolar liquid in the foetal lamb.* Journal of Physiology, London, **204**, 159–168.
2. Battaglia, F.C., Meschia, G., Hellegers, A.E. and Barron, D.H. (1958). *The effects of acute hypoxia on the osmotic pressure of the plasma.* Quarterly Journal of Experimental Physiology **43**, 197–208.
3. Battaglia, F.C., Prystowsky, H., Smisson, C., Hellegers, A. and Bruns, P.D. (1960). *Fetal blood studies. XIII. The effect of the administration of fluids intravenously to mothers upon the concentrations of water and electrolytes in plasma of human fetuses.* Pediatrics **25**, 2–10.
4. Baum, J.D., Eisenberg, C., Franklin, F.A. Jr., Meschia, G. and Battaglia, F.C. (1971). *Studies on colloid osmotic pressure in the fetus and newborn infant.* Biology of the Neonate **18**, 311–320.
5. Boyd, R.D.H., Haworth, C., Stacey, T.E. and Ward, R.H.T. (1976). *Permeability of the sheep placenta to unmetabolized polar nonelectrolytes.* Journal of Physiology **256**, 617–634.
6. Boyd, R.D.H., Stacey, T.E., Ward, R.H.T. and Weedon, A.P. (1978). *The sheep placenta as an epithelium.* In "Fetal and Newborn Cardiovascular Physiology" (L.D. Longo and D.D. Reneau, eds.), Volume 2, pp 449–474, Garland STPM Press, New York.
7. Bruns, P.D., Linder, R.O., Drose, V.E. and Battaglia, F.C. (1963). *The placental transfer of water from fetus to mother following the intravenous infusion of hypertonic mannitol to the maternal rabbit.* American Journal of Obstetrics and Gynecology **86**, 160–166.

8. Bruns, P.D., Hellegers, A.E., Seeds, A.E. Jr., Behrman, R.E. and Battaglia, F.C. (1964). *Effects of osmotic gradients across the primate placenta upon fetal and placental water contents.* Pediatrics **34**, 407–411.

9. Clements, J.A. and Tooley, W.H. (1977). *Kinetics of surface-active material in fetal lung.* In "Development of the Lung. Lung Biology in Health and Disease," (W.A. Hodson, ed.), Volume 6, pp 349–366, Marcel Dekker, Inc., New York.

10. Cloete, J.H.L. (1939). "Prenatal Growth in the Merino Sheep," Thesis, Onderstepoort Journal of Veterinary Science and Animal Industry, Volume 13, Number 2, pp 418–548, Government Printer, Pretoria, South Africa.

10a. Davson, H. (1956). "Physiology of the Ocular and Cerebral Fluids." Churchill Livingstone, London.

11. Delivoria-Papadopoulos, M., Battaglia, F.C. and Meschia, G. (1969). *A comparison of fetal versus maternal plasma colloidal osmotic pressure in man.* Proceedings of the Society for Experimental Biology and Medicine **131**, 84–87.

12. Faber, J.J. and Thornburg, K.L. (1983). *Placental reflection coefficients and filtration of water.* In "Placental Physiology. Structure and Function of Fetomaternal Exchange," (J.J. Faber and K.L. Thornburg, eds.), pp 91–96, Raven Press, New York.

13. Gresham, E.L., Rankin, J.H.G., Makowski, E.L., Meschia, G. and Battaglia, F.C. (1972). *An evaluation of fetal renal function in a chronic sheep preparation.* Journal of Clinical Investigation **51**, 149–156.

14. Hallman, M., Kulovich, M.V., Kirkpatrick, E., Sugarman, R.G. and Gluck, L. (1976). *Phosphatidylinositol and phosphatidylglycerol in amniotic fluid: Indices of lung maturity.* American Journal of Obstetrics and Gynecology **125**, 613–617.

15. Hutchinson, D.L., Gray, M.J., Plentl, A.A., Alvarez, H., Caldeyro-Barcia, R., Kaplan, B. and Lind, J. (1959). *The role of the fetus in the water exchange of the amniotic fluid of normal and hydramniotic patients.* Journal of Clinical Investigation **38**, 971–980.

16. Jacque, L. (1902). *De la Genère liquides amniotique et allantoidien. Cyroscopie et analyses chimiques.* Archives of International Physiology **3**, 463–469.

17. Jobe, A. (1984). *Fetal lung maturation and the respiratory distress syndrome. In* "Fetal Physiology and Medicine. The Basis of Perinatology," (R.W. Beard and P.W. Nathanielsz, eds.), Second Edition, pp 317–351, Marcel Dekker, Inc., New York.

18. Jost, A. and Policard, A. (1948). *Contribution expérimentale à l'étude du développement prénatal du poumon chez le lapin.* Archives of Anatomy and Microbiology **37**, 323.

19. Lumbers, E.R., Smith, F.G. and Stevens, A.D. (1985). *Measurement of net transplacental transfer of fluid to the fetal sheep.* Journal of Physiology **364**, 289–299.

20. Mellor, D.J. and Slater, J.S. (1972). *Daily changes in foetal urine and relationships with amniotic and allantoic fluid and maternal plasma during the last two months of pregnancy in conscious, unstressed ewes with chronically implanted catheters.* Journal of Physiology **227**, 503–525.

21. Meschia, G. (1955). *Colloidal osmotic pressures of fetal and maternal plasmas of sheep and goats.* American Journal of Physiology **181**, 1–8.

22. Meschia, G., Battaglia, F.C. and Barron, D.H. (1957). *A comparison of the freezing points of fetal and maternal plasmas of sheep and goat.* Quarterly Journal of Experimental Physiology **42**, 163–170.

23. Needham, G. (1931). "Chemical Embryology," The Macmillan Company, New York.

24. Olver, R.E. (1977). *Solute and water transfer in fetal and newborn lungs. In* "Development of the Lung," (W.A. Hodson, ed.), pp 525–559, Marcel Dekker, Inc., New York.

25. Strang, L.B. (1977). "Neonatal Respiration—Physiological and Clinical Studies." Blackwell Scientific Publications, Oxford.

26. Wladimiroff, J.W. and Campbell, S. (1974). *Fetal urine production rates in normal and complicated pregnancy.* Lancet **1**, 151–154.

Index

Letters *f* and *t* following page numbers refer to figures and tables.